HEALTHY BONES

D0249159

About the Author

Dr. Nancy Appleton received her Ph.D. in clinical nutrition. She is a nutritionist with a private practice in the Los Angeles area. She lectures extensively throughout the United States and Canada, and has appeared on numerous television and radio shows. She is the author of the bestseller, *Lick the Sugar Habit*.

HEALTHY BONES

WHAT YOU SHOULD KNOW ABOUT OSTEOPOROSIS

NANCY APPLETON, Ph.D.

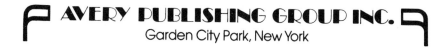
AVERY PUBLISHING GROUP INC.
Garden City Park, New York

The health procedures and opinions in this book are based on the training, personal experiences, and research of the author. Because each person and situation is unique, the editor and the publisher urge the reader to check with a qualified health professional before using any procedure where there is any question as to its appropriateness.

The publisher does not advocate the use of any particular diet, but believes the information presented in this book should be available to the public.

Because there is always some risk involved, the author and publisher are not responsible for any adverse effects or consequences resulting from the use of any of the suggestions, preparations, or procedures in this book. Please do not use the book if you are unwilling to assume the risk. Feel free to consult a physician or other qualified health professional. It is a sign of wisdom, not cowardice, to seek a second or third opinion.

Cover Design: Rudy Shur and Janine Eisner-Wall
In-House Editor: Marie Caratozzolo
Typesetter: Straight Creek Company, Denver, Colorado

Library of Congress Cataloging-in-Publication Data

Appleton, Nancy
    Healthy bones / Nancy Appleton.
      p. cm.
    Includes bibliographical references and index.
    ISBN 0-89529-462-1
    1. Osteoporosis—Prevention. 2. Osteoporosis—Diet therapy—
Recipes. I. Title.
RC931.073A66 1991
616.7' 16—dc20

Copyright © 1991 Nancy Appleton

All rights reserved. No part of this publication may be reproduced, stored in a retrieval system, or transmitted, in any form or by any means, electronic, mechanical, photocopying, recording or otherwise, without the prior written permission of the copyright owner.

Printed in the United States of America

10   9   8   7   6   5   4   3   2

Contents

Preface

Healthy Bones was written because I felt the public was really in the dark when it came to the available information on osteoporosis. The average person believes that taking extra calcium will prevent osteoporosis. *Healthy Bones* shows that taking extra calcium can actually make that calcium toxic to the body; extra calcium can deplete other minerals, as well. This book also describes how each one of us creates his own osteoporosis by making the calcium in our bodies unavailable for our bones!

The first part of this book explains what osteoporosis is, who gets it, and what the causes are. What follows next is a short discussion of our body chemistry, the functions of the endocrine system, and how a malfunctioning of our body system can cause osteoporosis. Our twentieth century lifestyle is discussed, as well as ways to keep it from affecting our health. Finally, the last part of the book provides practical lifestyle information: food plans, healthy eating suggestions, and recipes, all presented so the reader can follow a program to prevent or arrest osteoporosis.

I offer *Healthy Bones* with the sincerest desire to show what people can do to arrest the insidious condition of osteoporosis, and to provide the tools to prevent its manifestation.

Nancy Appleton, Ph.D.

1 | Holey Bones

Osteoporosis is an American epidemic! Just consider these statistics:

- In the United States, among people 60 years old, 35 percent of the women and 10 percent of the men have osteoporosis.
- By 70 years of age, 50 percent of all women have brittle bones.
- Osteoporosis is the cause of 90 percent of all fractures after the age of 65.
- In women over 65 years old, 50 percent have bone mineral density below the fracture threshold.
- The average American loses $1^1/_2$ inches of height each decade after menopause as a result of vertebral collapse.
- Among those suffering from osteoporosis, 14 percent will die as the result of broken hips.

- Over a million fractures a year are caused by osteoporosis.
- At least 40 percent of all people over 60 years of age have lost their teeth to periodontal disease (osteoporosis of the mouth).
- Osteoporosis is the most common systemic bone disorder in the United States. It affects 15 million people, primarily women, causing thousands of injuries and deaths per year.
- Over $1 billion a year is spent on treating conditions related to osteoporosis.

What is this disease and what causes it?

What is Osteoporosis?

Literally, osteoporosis means "porous bones"; it is a weakening condition of the bones that results in a slow, insidious loss of calcium. When calcium is pulled from the bones, the amount of bone is reduced and the strength of the remaining bone is severely weakened. Osteoporosis can be regarded as the condition that exists when bone mass has been reduced to such an extent that the skeleton becomes vulnerable to fractures arising from minor falls or the stresses of daily activities. One might do something as simple as bend over to tie a shoe or step down some stairs, and a fracture will occur.

Osteoporosis is a degenerative disease that starts slowly. For some, it can take hold as early as childhood. For others, it develops in adulthood. In women, it can accelerate after menopause. In men, it accelerates after age 65.

Unlike other bone diseases, osteoporosis is not associated with abnormal bone composition. The bones of osteoporotic people are no different than normal bones. There is simply less of the bone.

Who Develops Osteoporosis?

Those most likely to be afflicted by osteoporosis are postmenopausal women who are Caucasian and of Northern European descent. Others, whose chance for osteoporosis is high, are fair-skinned, petite women; those who smoke; those who drink alcohol and/or coffee; those who take antacids, corticosteroids, or antibiotics; those who do not exercise, are paralyzed, or are bedridden; those who have a history of osteoporosis in their families; and those who have experienced early menopause, whether naturally or through a hysterectomy.

Thin people are more prone to osteoporosis than obese people because overweight people have fat cells, which can turn a hormone secreted by the adrenal gland into estrogen. The more estrogen we have, the less likely we are to get osteoporosis. Men are less likely to get osteoporosis because they start with a larger bone mass and do not go through the drastic hormonal changes that women face during menstruation and menopause. Black women develop osteoporosis less often because their bones are generally denser to begin with, and it, therefore, takes longer to reach the levels of loss that lead to fractures and disabling pains. Anorexic women, regardless of age, are more prone to osteoporosis. They continually upset their body chemistries due to stress, not eating correctly, and not eating enough.

What are the Symptoms of Osteoporosis?

Osteoporosis affects the body in many different ways. The main symptom is a loss of height due to the compression of weakened vertebrae. Other symptoms may include:

- cramps in the legs and feet at night
- bone pain
- lower back pain
- fractures of the hips, spine, wrists, or other parts of the skeleton
- dowager's hump, a forward bending of the spine
- extreme fatigue
- excess plaque on the teeth
- periodontal disease
- rickets
- brittle or soft fingernails
- premature grey hair
- heart palpitations

What Causes Osteoporosis?

My thesis is that an upset body chemistry is the cause of osteoporosis. When our body chemistries are in balance (homeostasis) over decades, we will not get osteoporosis. When our body chemistries are upset continually, when we cannot maintain homeostasis, we are more likely to get degenerative diseases. One of these diseases is osteoporosis.

Our bones are continually undergoing a process of remodeling. This process involves bone reabsorption, where minerals are removed from the bones, and bone formation, where minerals are put back into the bones. Osteoporosis occurs when there is too much bone reabsorption and not enough bone formation. The reason that there is not enough bone formation is that we upset our body chemistries. This can cause calcium to be pulled from the bones in order to maintain a calcium homeostasis in the blood.

This is by no means an irreversible process. The key to stopping osteoporosis lies in a balanced body chemistry and a delicate balance of minerals in the blood that helps the body function optimally.

In the chapters that follow, we will take a look at homeostasis, how the body chemistry works, what happens when it is disrupted, and the culprits that cause the disruption. You'll have a complete plan for returning the body to balance and ridding it of the danger of osteoporosis.

Osteoporosis is completely preventable without drugs, without extensive supplements, and without expensive treatments. Once you know how to return your body to its homeostatic balance, osteoporosis can be prevented or arrested. Amazingly, other symptoms such as headaches, arthritis, and skin disorders will also disappear.

2 | Your Body Chemistry

When all the minerals, hormones, pH, and other elements that make up the body's internal chemistry are in perfect balance, the body is said to be in homeostasis. When the body is in homeostasis, the pH (acid/alkaline) balance is correct, the minerals are balanced with each other, the endocrine glands secrete the right amount of hormones into the bloodstream, and the body hums along. This state of balance encourages proper performance of those internal functions necessary for growth, healing, and life itself. These include the regulation of mineral ratios, the production of enzymes, and the total digestive process.

With an upset body chemistry, the pH becomes either too acidic or too alkaline, the mineral relationships become upset, and the endocrine glands secrete too much (or not enough) of their hormones. The body no longer hums, but honks, now and then, with symptoms such as fatigue, joint pains, headaches, or low blood sugar. The body has many mechanisms designed to maintain homeostasis, because only when the body chemistry is balanced can the body work efficiently.

Please refer to Figure 2.1 as I take you on a tour of the various glands in our wonderfully designed bodies. These glands can contribute to or be detrimental to homeostasis.

The Endocrine System

The endocrine glands, which are scattered throughout the body, secrete hormones into the bloodstream and help regulate the body chemistry. Each of these glands—the adrenals, pancreas, thyroid, parathyroid, pituitary, and gonads—plays an important part in maintaining homeostasis.

Whenever we upset our body chemistries, a chain reaction occurs among these guardians of homeostasis. As they try to bring balance back to the bloodstream, they often pull calcium and other minerals from the bones. When this happens repeatedly, over years of upset body chemistry, osteoporosis is a likely result.

The Adrenal Glands

Back in primitive times, when cave men and women were being chased by bears, they went into a "fight/flight" syndrome—either stay and fight the bear or run out of the bear's way. At a critical time like this, the adrenal glands would secrete adrenalin into the bloodstream to provide the necessary added energy.

Today, although we're not likely to encounter bears on a regular basis, the "fight/flight" function of the adrenals remains. They secrete adrenalin whenever the stress in our lives

FIGURE 2.1

THE ENDOCRINE SYSTEM

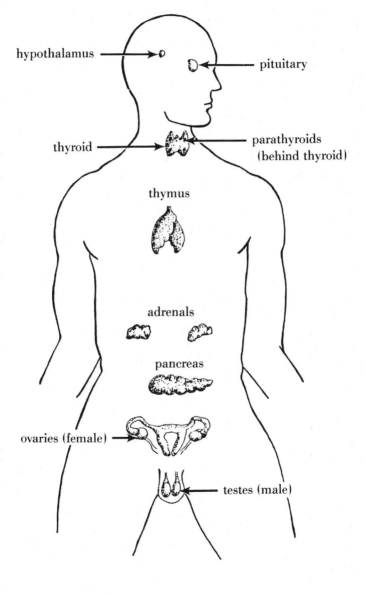

hypothalamus

pituitary

thyroid

parathyroids
(behind thyroid)

thymus

adrenals

pancreas

ovaries (female)

testes (male)

becomes distress. This stress usually manifests itself in terms of anger, depression, feelings of resentment toward others, and so on. I hate to tell all those coffee-loving people out there, but coffee can also stimulate the adrenals into action.

Since adrenalin is capable of dissolving bone, overactive adrenal glands can play havoc with the skeletal system. The adrenal glands slow down their production of bone-dissolving hormones around your 65th birthday, which could be a reason why bone loss decreases at this time.

The Pancreas

When table sugar, fruit, or other simple sugars are eaten, the blood glucose (sugar) level rises. The pancreas secretes a hormone called insulin into the bloodstream, and the blood sugar level returns to normal. This is a normal homeostatic mechanism.

When we eat too much simple sugar or upset our body chemistries in other ways, the pancreas can begin to malfunction. It can secrete too much or too little insulin. If the pancreas does not secrete enough insulin, the result is high blood sugar (hyperglycemia), or diabetes. If the pancreas secretes too much insulin, the result is low blood sugar (hypoglycemia).

The Thyroid

Thyroxine, the thyroid hormone, regulates metabolic function in the body. Most tissues are stimulated by the thyroid hormone, especially the liver and the muscles. When thyroid secretion is excessive, the condition is called *hyper*thyroidism.

Hyperthyroid individuals have an overactive thyroid and an elevated basal metabolic rate. They tend to be hyperactive, produce more body heat, and burn their food at higher rates than normal individuals.

*Hypo*thyroidism is a condition characterized by an underactive thyroid and a lowered basal metabolic rate. People with this condition tend to be sluggish, produce a lower rate of body heat, and burn food at a slower rate. They tend to be overweight.

Too little thyroxine in childhood can lead to stunted growth, while a deficiency as an adult can cause bone pain and spontaneous fractures. If thyroxine becomes excessive in the bloodstream, it can increase the rate of bone turnover (the wearing away of calcium in the bones) because of its ability to increase the body's metabolic rate, thereby mobilizing calcium stores. This can result in calcium excretion in the urine and can also raise the level of calcium in the blood, upsetting the homeostasis of the body and removing calcium from the bones.

It is interesting to note that Dr. B. Ettinger's research shows that women taking supplements equivalent to or greater than three grains of dessicated thyroid had significantly lower bone mass than women who did not take the thyroid hormone. If you take a thyroid hormone, have your blood tested periodically by a qualified health practitioner to make sure you are taking the minimum dose for maximum effect.

The Parathyroid Glands

These four small glands, located in the neck at the base of the thyroid gland, are the calcium regulators. They regulate the amount of calcium secreted into the bloodstream, reserved in the bones, or excreted from the body. If the calcium in the blood should fall below critical levels, the glands release a hormone called *parathormone* (PTH). Parathormone does the following:

- signals the kidneys to put calcium back into the bloodstream, rather than excreting it from the body through the urine
- stimulates the conversion of Vitamin D from an inactive to an active form, thereby allowing the intestines to absorb more calcium from the foods we eat
- stimulates the breakdown of bone, which, in turn, releases stored calcium into the bloodstream

Calcium is so critical to life that the body is willing to sacrifice bone mass to ensure adequate levels of calcium in the bloodstream. When there is excess calcium in the bloodstream, the parathyroid glands help to put the calcium back into the bones. There is a continual small "push-pull" going on all the time, all part of the homeostatic mechanisms.

If the parathyroids malfunction, due to upset body chemistry, and secrete too much or not enough of their hormones, extra calcium can be pulled from the bones and tissues, severely weakening them. When parathormone is released into the bloodstream, a signal is given to the kidneys to send calcium back into the bloodstream instead of secreting it into the urine.

PTH is stimulated by phosphorus. When excess phosphorus is put into the bloodstream, due to upset body chemistry, the blood wants to maintain a calcium to phosphorus ratio of 2.5 to 1. Therefore, it will pull calcium out of the bones in order to maintain that balance. An overactive parathyroid gland can be a problem. Estrogen has the ability to block the activity of the PTH, but estrogen can also be blocked by upset body chemistry.

The Pituitary Gland

There are actually two parts of the pituitary gland, the anterior pituitary and the posterior pituitary; they are considered separate glands. One of the things the anterior pituitary does is secrete a hormone that controls growth. An underactive anterior pituitary may lead to dwarfism. Conversely, if the anterior pituitary gland is very much overactive in its production of growth hormone, the result is a giant. More research still needs to be done on this hormone in order to understand its effects on bone.

The post pituitary gland secretes hormones that help control the salt and water balance of the body and the gravity and density of the urine. If this gland is not functioning well, a person might have to urinate more often. If you have to get up in the night to urinate, one of your homeostatic mechanisms might not be functioning optimally.

The Gonads

The gonads secrete the male and female hormones, which play a role in balanced body chemistry. The male sex glands, known as testes, produce the male hormone testosterone. Both males and females produce this hormone, but males produce more than females. Ovaries, the female sex glands, produce estrogen and progesterone. Males also produce these hormones in minute amounts. Estrogen stimulates the liver to produce a protein that binds to certain adrenal hormones, lessening their ability to dissolve bone.

There is evidence that deficiencies in certain hormones may lead to bone loss. A deficiency in estrogen may contribute to bone loss after menopause. And yet, there is very little osteoporosis among the Bantu women of Africa, even after menopause, which occurs at the same age as American women. Studies show that post-menopausal Bantu women have more estrogen than post-menopausal American women.

Why would the Bantu women have more estrogen than American women? Could it be that due to the American woman's twentieth century lifestyle she has upset her body chemistry more? As she ages, her hormones do not function as well.

Bantu women eat their native foods with a minimum of milk, no calcium supplements, and no estrogen pills after menopause. Also, they take in little sugar, caffeine, alcohol, aspirin, corticosteroids, antibiotics, or other drugs. The body stays in homeostasis much of the time and is not continually pulling calcium out of the bones over a lifetime. It would be interesting to test the post-menopausal Bantu women for thyroid function and other endocrine gland functions to see if other glands functioned better than American women's.

Another valuable study showed that 55 percent of post-menopausal women who did not have osteoporosis had insufficient calcium absorption to maintain a calcium balance, even though their diet included 872 milligrams of calcium per day. These researchers went on to say that taking more calcium would improve the balance. I don't necessarily agree with the conclusions found in this study because the only things controlled were the amounts of calcium, phosphorus, and protein. These subjects could have been consuming five cups of coffee, three candy bars, and a milkshake each day. Again, it all goes back to estrogen and why we have less than Bantu women, and probably all primitive women. The answer lies in our contemporary lifestyle with a big emphasis on diet.

All of our glands work in relation to one another. Without estrogen, certain glands cannot function well, but with too much estrogen, other glands may be disturbed. Estrogen can step up the growth of abnormal cancer cells. Birth control pills, which contain estrogen, may be incompatible with your health history, especially if you have had a liver tumor or breast cancer. Other women who might risk their health by taking estrogen are diabetics and smokers; women with cardiovascular problems, high blood pressure, elevated cholesterol levels; and those who have a family history of early cardiovascular trouble.

In 1968, the low-dose estrogen birth control pill was introduced. In terms of heart disease, it has helped to reduce the number of women developing venous thrombosis (blood clotting in the veins), but has had no effect on disease of the arteries or the overall death rate. In other words, women on the low-dose pill are still at an increased risk of dying from circulatory disease.

In the medical journal *Lancet*, the Royal College of General Practitioners revealed that women who have used the pill have a 40 percent higher death rate, mostly from circulatory disease. In 1977, a study of women using different methods of birth control showed that hospital admission rates for self-poisoning were twice as high for pill users as for women fitted with uterine devices, and four times higher than for women using the diaphragm.

Despite reports that the pill protects against breast cancer, there are more deaths from breast cancer among women on the pill than not on the pill. If you smoke and take the pill, there is a stronger chance that you will get cardiovascular disease. Both the pill and smoking suppress natural hormone functions. After years of this insult to the body, there is a further insult after menopause of hormone replacement therapy. Estrogen is given once more, but to an even more vulnerable age group.

All of the hormones secreted by the endocrine glands serve as regulatory mechanisms to keep the body chemistry in balance, to maintain homeostasis. Under normal circumstances, the chemical makeup of our blood fluctuates within a narrow range. The blood glucose level rises and falls a little. The amount of calcium in the blood goes up and down very slightly. All of the different chemicals in the body fluctuate within a very narrow range when the body is healthy. The minerals, enzymes, and hormones in the bloodstream can work together only when the body mechanisms are working correctly to maintain homeostasis.

Mineral Relationships

Figure 2.2 illustrates the minerals found in the bloodstream and how they relate to one another. Calcium and phosphorus, the most important minerals in our study of osteoporosis, work best in a 2.5 to 1 ratio. Normally, the calcium level in the bloodstream is about 10 milligrams per deciliter, and the phosphorus level is 4 milligrams. No matter what amount of calcium is present in the bloodstream, only the amount that is 2.5 times the phosphorus level can function optimally.

For example, if the phosphorus level is only 3 milligrams per deciliter, rather than the normal 4, only 7.5 milligrams of calcium will be able to function in the body. This is because the ratio must be 2.5 times the calcium to phosphorus for the minerals to function optimally. The rest will be secreted into the urine or may form hard deposits in soft tissue. Conversely, if there are only 5 milligrams of calcium, then only 2 milligrams of phosphorus will be able to function.

Copper and zinc are two other minerals that work in direct relation to each other. If the zinc becomes deficient, the copper can become toxic and vice versa. This is true of all the different minerals in the body; they all work in relation to one another. Therefore, directly or indirectly, all of the minerals can be affected if one of them becomes deficient or excessive. One of the first effects of an unbalanced body chemistry is a disruption of mineral relationships in the bloodstream. Some minerals become depleted while others become excessive.

When the body chemistry is upset, the amount of calcium can increase in the blood while the phosphorus level can de-

FIGURE 2.2

MINERAL WHEEL

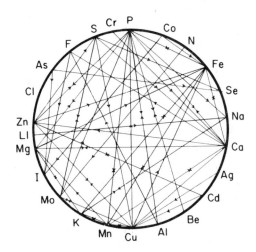

SOURCE: Dr. Paul Eck. Analytical Research Labs, Inc. Phoenix, Arizona.

crease, changing the all-important calcium-phosphorus ratio. If, for example, the calcium rises to 11 milligrams per deciliter, and the phosphorus drops to 3 milligrams per deciliter, the ratio is not 2.5 to 1, but closer to 3.5 to 1.

Calcium is best used by the body if it exists in a 2.5 to 1 ratio with the phosphorous. Therefore, even if there are 11 milligrams per deciliter in the blood, the body can only use 7.5 milligrams, or 2.5 times the 3 milligrams of phosphorus. If the phosphorus drops, so does the functioning calcium in the same ratio. Therefore, if phosphorus becomes depleted, calcium becomes depleted as well, whether it exists in the bloodstream or not.

There is an interesting phenomenon that takes place when calcium is pulled into the bloodstream from the bones.

In order to get into the bloodstream, calcium has to cross cell membranes. The only way it can cross over is with protein. Therefore, protein is pulled out of the bones and tissues whenever calcium is. This process has implications for other problems in the body such as lower back pain, as well as osteoporosis.

Tissues can become weak when protein is taken out of them. As a result, bones can shift out of alignment because the tissues are not strong enough to hold them into place. The slightest provocation can cause injury. A disk can rarify and become spongy, requiring surgical removal. A fall can break a hip. Leaning over to tie a shoe can result in a pinched nerve and inflammation can set in; the body may not heal, so a doctor might be forced to use drugs, such as cortisone. Cortisone is used to reduce inflammation, but is also known to draw calcium from the bones.

Our bodies are wonderful mechanisms. When they are treated well, with the right foods and a minimum amount of distress, homeostasis can be maintained on a continual basis. When our bodies are constantly bombarded with abusive foods and distress, homeostasis cannot be maintained. When this occurs, all of the minerals change in relation to each other, and some can become toxic while others can become deficient. The main minerals of concern in osteoporosis are calcium and phosphorus. Deficiencies and toxicities of other minerals are implicated in other diseases. Therefore, you can have osteoporosis and other diseases at the same time.

Acid/Alkaline Balance

The pH (acid/alkaline) balance of the body is another important indicator of homeostasis. When we digest foods, we form an ash as an end product. Some foods, such as animal protein, dairy products, eggs, and grains, form an acid ash. Other foods, such as fruits and vegetables, form an alkaline ash. Psychological distress, as well as sugar and processed or synthetic foods leave no ash, but have an acidifying effect on the body.

The pH must stay within a very narrow range for homeostasis to be maintained. The circulatory system—the blood system—serves all the other systems of the body, including the immune, nervous, digestive, and the respiratory systems. When the pH of the blood is balanced, the other systems in the body function well. The blood has developed a buffer system to keep the blood pH level at 7.4. When the pH becomes too acidic or too alkaline, one of the ways to regain homeostasis is through the buffer system.

Sodium is the first buffer to help bring an acidic pH back to balance. This is the sodium that is found in fruits and vegetables. It is loosely covalently bonded and easily utilized by the body. Table salt, which is actually sodium chloride, is a strong ionically bonded mineral and will not replenish the sodium needed for our buffer system. This salt resists being separated into the sodium and chloride ions that are usable by the body. Therefore, table salt is not a substitute for vegetables and fruits. Eating too much salt can actually pull calcium from the bones.

When the body is continually upset, the sodium becomes depleted. When sodium can no longer adequately buffer accumulated acid, the body uses calcium as a second buffer. Because of our twentieth century lifestyle, we are continually calling our buffer systems into action. The demand for calcium, for our buffer systems alone, contributes more to the depletion of calcium from the bones than does a deficiency of calcium intake. The 800 milligrams of daily calcium, recommended by the National Academy of Sciences, are not sufficient in preventing the extraction of calcium from the bones, as long as calcium is needed as a buffer to regain an alkaline pH and homeostasis. No amount of calcium will.

Dr. Amnon Wackman and Dr. Daniel Berstein from Harvard University have suggested that the increased incidence of osteoporosis with age may, in part, be the result of a lifelong utilization of the body's buffering capacity for the constant balancing of pH homeostasis. When there is a constant assault on this buffering process, the bones lose their minerals and osteoporosis is a natural result.

Our bodies have evolved over hundreds of thousands of years. Our biochemistry is essentially the same as it was several hundred thousand years ago. While these biochemical pathways and biological processes were evolving, the lifestyle of the day set the precedent. It determined how much calcium our system could make for the buffer system, and how much change the pH system was geared to handle. But primitive man did not have access to the refined, overcooked foods that modern man does, foods that are difficult to digest and that overload the metabolic pathways.

Today, the average person eats, thinks, and lives in such a way that these metabolic pathways become exhausted. The blood becomes acidic, calcium is excreted into the urine, all of the minerals become upset, and enzymes can't function. It is metabolic overload that exhausts our buffer systems and causes the loss of calcium that leads to osteoporosis.

Enzymes

Enzymes are chemical catalysts that trigger reactions in the body. They make things happen, but don't change themselves. Almost all enzymes depend on minerals in order to function. Any disruption in mineral levels will cause a disruption in the enzymes' abilities to do their jobs. There are two types of enzymes: metabolic enzymes and digestive enzymes.

Metabolic enzymes help with the tissues and organs in the body. They do the special work needed to run the heart, brain, lungs, kidneys, and other organs. Although thousands of enzymes are known, many more reactions have been identified in which the enzymes responsible are not yet recognized. Hundreds of metabolic enzymes are necessary to carry on the work in the body, to repair damage, to remove decay, and to help the healing process.

Digestive enzymes help break food down into its simplest components. Lipase, a fat-digesting enzyme, helps reduce fats to fatty acids. Amylase helps change carbohydrates into simple sugars, and protein is converted into amino acids by protease.

Normally, when we put food into our mouths and it goes along the digestive path, enzymes are secreted from the lining of the gastro-intestinal tract. These enzymes help break down the food into its smallest components. When the food has been broken down into fatty acids, simple sugars, and amino acids, it is taken into the bloodstream by *villi*—wavy, finger-like projections that line the gastro-intestinal tract. The cells then get the nutrients, vitamins, minerals, amino acids, fatty acids, and simple sugars they need to build and repair themselves. Healthy, happy bodies are the result.

But when the digestive enzymes cannot function optimally, due to upset body chemistry and the depletion of minerals, all of the food does not digest. Some of it seems to putrify in the gut, irritating the lining of the intestinal tract and causing the cells of the lining to widen. This is called the *leaky gut syndrome*. The undigested, or partially digested, food gets into the bloodstream where it doesn't belong. This food cannot be utilized by the cells because it is too large; it hasn't been broken down to its simplest form.

Instead, it swims around in the bloodstream causing havoc in the body. This undigested food in the bloodstream is a form of allergy. It can cause such classic allergic symptoms as runny eyes and noses, scratchy throats, itchy ears, sneezes and wheezes, headaches, fatigue, and dizziness. It can affect the joints by causing arthritis. It can attack the skin and cause swelling, psoriasis, and rashes or other skin problems. The immune system, which protects the body from foreign invaders such as bacteria and viruses, looks at this undigested food as a foreign invader and reacts accordingly.

The immune system must come to the defense of our bodies and remove the undigested food from the bloodstream. Unfortunately, our immune systems were not meant to do this every time we upset our body chemistries by our lifestyle. Our immune systems will become exhausted. This exhaustion of the immune system is part of the *degenerative disease process*.

Lack of Homeostasis and Osteoporosis

A body that is continually out of homeostasis is a body that is slowly on the road to degenerative disease. For some people, osteoporosis is the result. The simple reason so many people are getting osteoporosis is that they spend a great deal of time out of homeostasis. When a body is out of homeostasis and its mineral balance becomes upset, the calcium becomes deficient. A body with upset body chemistry is prone to brittle bones.

In terms of osteoporosis, the parathyroid gland should be functioning as well as possible at all times, since this gland regulates the amount of calcium in the bloodstream. With the continual insult to the body by our twentieth-century lifestyle, the parathyroid gland stops functioning optimally and cannot effectively regulate the calcium and phosphorus levels.

Osteoporosis can develop out of a continual drop in either calcium or phosphorus. If the phosphorus drops, there might be plenty of calcium in the blood, but it cannot function effectively. Since calcium can only function in relation to phosphorus, the parathyroid gland may react to a lack of functioning calcium in the bloodstream by pulling calcium from the bones and tissues.

Other Diseases

Osteoporosis is not the only calcium-related disease. Many people continually upset their body chemistries, but do not get osteoporosis. In fact, the diseases people get are largely determined by genetic blueprint. The diseases of parents and grandparents and the genetic weaknesses in ones body influence what disease will result when homeostasis can no longer be maintained. It could be cancer, heart disease, multiple sclerosis, or any other disease. Following are a few diseases that are directly related to osteoporosis.

Osteomalacia

Osteomalacia is the adult equivalency of rickets. It is a deficiency of calcium and phosphorus crystals in the collagen framework of the bone. It can be a forewarning of osteoporosis.

A connection has been found between osteomalacia and Vitamin D. Samuel H. Doppelt and associates at Massachusetts General Hospital in Boston checked 142 elderly patients with hip fractures for Vitamin D levels. They found all of the levels of Vitamin D to be low. Of these patients, 75 percent had osteomalacia.

Vitamin D is needed to assure the assimilation of calcium, phosphorus, and magnesium. Cholesterol and sunlight work together to form Vitamin D in the skin. So, a diet too low (or too high) in cholesterol can be a problem. Without sufficient cholesterol, it is difficult for the body to assimilate fat-soluble vitamins such as A, E, and D.

Periodontal Disease

Periodontal disease includes everything that can happen in those parts of the mouth that surround the teeth. Other names for periodontal disease are pyorrhea, gum disorders, and osteoporosis of the mouth.

In a study of white women between the ages of 60 and 69, a definite correlation was found between tooth loss and bone loss elsewhere in the body. Women with reduced cortical bone (the hard dense bone that forms the outer shell of all bones) in the fingers were more likely to have full or partial dentures than women with more cortical bone.

As the jawbone becomes more porous and therefore weaker, the teeth are less firmly anchored. They start shifting around. The gums become inflamed and the periodontal bone recedes. Bacteria are then free to invade the open pockets between the gums and teeth.

We all breathe bacteria into our mouths. Bacteria alone do not cause periodontal disease, but they do work in relationship with inflamed gums and receding periodontal bones to cause periodontal disease.

ZIGGY

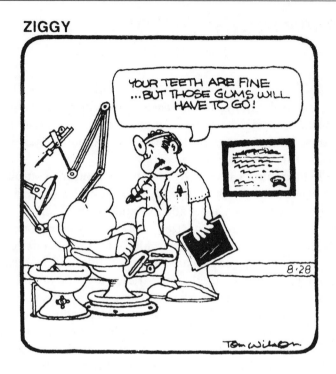

Ziggy © 1989 Ziggy and Friends. Distributed by Universal Press Syndicate. Reprinted with permission. All rights reserved.

Diabetes

There is direct evidence showing that diabetics have a reduced amount of bone. Dr. Toni McCain believes that when the sugar level gets too high in the blood of diabetics, it depresses the calcium absorption in the gut.

Diabetics of both sexes have significantly more osteoporosis than those in age-matched control groups. This osteoporosis can manifest itself in vertebral and neck fractures, or any other kind of fracture.

Osteoarthritis

The main joints of the body are the ankles, knees, hips, shoulders, and elbows. If they seem to be chronically stiff or make strange noises when you move them, you might be a candidate for osteoarthritis—arthritis of the bones and cartilage. But this doesn't have to be.

When you upset your body chemistry, immune complexes can collect in the joints. These immune complexes consist of an antigen, such as a food allergy, and an antibody, a substance our body makes to attack foreign invaders (such as bacteria, viruses, or undigested food) in the bloodstream. These immune complexes cause deterioration and fraying of the cartilage and tendons that are attached to the joints.

When we upset our body chemistry, we can create excess calcium in the blood. This excess, nonfunctioning, and toxic calcium is attracted to the joints, possibly in an attempt to reinforce the attachments. If functioning calcium is lacking in the blood, it will actually be removed from the bones and may be deposited in the weak joints. Large deposits of calcium in these joints make them difficult to move and cause a crippling inflammatory effect. This is known as arthritis.

If an arthritic fasts for three days on distilled or mineral water, all or most of the arthritic pain will go away. He will then be able to see the connection between the food he eats and the pain. Once he starts eating again, it is important to figure out what foods are upsetting him and he must remove those foods from his diet. (Fasting is NOT advisable for those arthritics who are taking drugs as the drugs need to be taken with food.) The arthritic must also deal with any stress in his life. A change in diet and lifestyle will free the arthritic from this inflammatory process and pain.

At the same time, a calcium deficiency is also created because not all of it can function due to the low phosphorus. This deficiency of calcium in the bloodstream causes the parathyroid gland to secrete a hormone that helps in getting some of the calcium from your bones into your blood. When this is done over a period of time, bones eventually lose minerals and become brittle and osteoporotic. You can become arthritic and osteoporotic at the same time, as well as having other health problems.

These are only a few of the diseases that can be caused by upset body chemistry. For some, the disease could be arthritis, multiple sclerosis, lupus, heart disease, or any other disease involving weakness of certain tissues. It is also possible to have more than one set of weakened or inflamed tissues. Many people have many symptoms throughout their bodies and have more than one disease.

We were all born with a genetic blueprint. We were born with certain weaknesses and certain strengths. We are not all born equal in terms of body chemistry. Some of us are genetically stronger than others. There is not much we can do about our genetic blueprints, but there is something we can do about our lifestyles.

Our genetic blueprints do not need to manifest themselves in terms of disease unless our body chemistries are continually upset. We do not have to get diseases. We do not need to get osteoporosis. We keep these diseases away by keeping our body chemistries in balance—in homeostasis.

Now let's take a look at some of the factors that cause the body chemistry to become upset.

3 | What's Eating You?

It is rarely just one factor that causes problems in the body, but many factors working together. It is possible to overdose on two or more different stressors. Perhaps you would be fine having a small piece of carrot cake. But if you also had a hamburger, milkshake, and french fries, and became angry at the waitress because she was slow in bringing your order, the combination of stressors could overload your body chemistry.

When this metabolic overload occurs, the body exhausts its buffer systems and can no longer maintain a normal pH. The enzymes can no longer function optimally. The body becomes compromised and, over a period of time, the degenerative disease process ensues.

In this chapter, the various stressors that can cause metabolic overload are discussed. You may be amazed when you discover how many different ways your body can be abused by today's modern lifestyle.

Mental and Physical Distress

Of all the factors that upset the body chemistry, change the mineral relationships, and cause calcium to become depleted, distress is the number one culprit. Not only does it cause alienation between people, but it also causes osteoporosis and other diseases.

We all have stress in our lives. We have parents, we have children, we drive on freeways, we work for a living. This is stress. It is not life's situations—the parents, children, freeways, and jobs—but how we view them and deal with them that determines whether they become distress. When we get angry, depressed, play victim, hold judgments against others, and try to get back at people, the stress in our lives becomes distress. It is this distress that causes problems, not the stress.

Mental distress may, in fact, be the key to the increasing prevalence of osteoporosis. Why is osteoporosis so much more prevalent today than at the turn of the century? I believe that our lifestyle has changed considerably in the past hundred years, and a great deal of distress has been added.

Back at the turn of the century, our eating habits were completely different from what they are today. Much of the food was grown on local farms, and people prepared the food themselves at home. Few chemicals were used when growing fruits and vegetables. Cattle roamed the range, as did chickens and pigs. The average person ate between twenty and thirty pounds of sugar per year. Soft drinks were unheard of, as were fast foods.

Our family units were more stable. It wasn't unusual for three generations to live together. In 1900, only 20 percent of all women worked outside the home, Men, too, were closer to home. Their jobs did not take them across continents. They didn't have to drive long distances to work. They were a much more integral part of the family.

Children had a better chance of growing up in the constant presence of people who loved them. There was always someone there from the family to bandage a scratched knee, read a book, rock them when they needed extra love, and listen to tales of their school adventures. When the parents weren't around, there were always grandparents to take their place.

Today, our eating habits are very different. Produce is shipped around the world according to the season. In the United States, we get lamb from New Zealand and strawberries from Australia. Foods are sprayed with insecticides, pesticides, and fungicides. Recently, the United States Government has allowed the radiation of some of our food. Cattle no longer graze, but are kept in pens. Chickens are often kept in indoor chicken coops and never see the light of day. Because of these conditions, farm animals get sick and need antibiotics continuously. Our cattle and poultry are not as healthy as they were at the turn of the century.

Today, we eat approximately 130 pounds of sugar, per person, per year. That is the equivalent of almost a half a cup per day. We drink an average of 482 soft drinks a year, per person, 380 of which contain sugar. The average person's diet is 42 percent fat, much of it from fried foods—potato chips, french fries, corn chips, fried chicken, fish and chips, fried hamburgers, fried eggs, and tempura. Our kitchen cupboards are filled with processed foods. Only a small portion of supermarket space is used for fresh fruits, vegetables, and meats; the rest is processed, packaged, or frozen.

Today's lifestyle lends itself to a fast-paced, "not-enough-hours-in-the-day" type of existence. When we eat, we lean toward foods that are quick to prepare and easy to eat. We buy fast food and eat it on the run, or gobble it down while reading about some disaster in the newspapers, watching a "shoot-em-up" on TV, or writing a report for work that was due yesterday. There is little time in our hectic day for cooking a meal from basics, so TV dinners, packaged spaghetti, and frozen or canned vegetables are the usual fare.

How we eat, where we eat, why we eat, and what we eat have all become confused. Nutritious food is no longer the number one priority. For many people, eating is a purely social activity. The main part of their social lives is meeting someone for a drink after work, inviting people over for drinks and dinner, getting together for a poker game with beer and chips, or meeting someone at a restaurant. The average working adult eats in a restaurant eleven times a week.

There is something about breaking bread with someone that makes them a special friend. Our social lives revolve around food and eating. We eat things because they taste good, look good, and smell good, not because they are good for us. Our taste buds have changed. Carrots no longer taste sweet because of all the excessively sweet things we eat. All these changes in our eating habits make a difference in our body chemistry, the way we feel, and the state of our health.

Families, too, have changed. Generally, grandparents no longer live with younger generations, but in senior communities and the like. Of all mothers with children under seventeen years of age, 71 percent now work outside of the home. Loving moments are not as prevalent for children, and often there is not much continuity in their lives. Divorce, and the anger and rage that accompanies it, plays a role. Children have more distress as they grow up, and many do not learn how to cope well with life's situations. They grow up into frustrated, angry, and bitter adults.

Knowingly and unknowingly, we create our own osteoporosis. Knowingly and unknowingly, we cause our own disease. It is up to each of us to deal with the stress in our lives and not let it become distress. We must learn to let go of frustrations, resentments, and anger. Just thinking an angry or depressing thought or holding a judgment against someone can cause minerals to be depleted or become toxic.

It's amazing what the mind can do. A twenty-nine-year-old man, with a history of psychosis, was admitted to a hospital complaining of severe chest pains and a burning and tingling sensation in the upper parts of his body. A blood test revealed his phosphorus to be very low. When the doctor reassured the patient that he was not dying of a heart attack, the phosphorus went right back to normal. The mind can actually change the minerals in the body for better or worse in a short period of time.

Physical pain, like mental pain, can upset the body chemistry. Severe burns can cause a depletion of phosphorus. When a person hyperventilates, phosphorus is depleted in the blood.

I was interested to discover what stress does to the body, so I had some volunteers arrive one morning after fasting for twelve hours. I took blood from each of them to find the calcium and phosphorus ratio. Then I immersed one of each of their hands in ice water, creating distress for their bodies. I took their blood right afterward and watched the calcium go up and the phosphorus go down. Whenever that ratio changes, all of the minerals become upset, and so does the body chemistry.

Physical pain can lead to mental pain. Mental pain can lead to physical pain. The mind/body connection becomes clearer each day. Distress can upset the body chemistry and lead to allergies. Allergies can upset the body and lead to severe stress.

An operation, a car accident, over-exercising, being exposed to too much heat or too much cold can all upset the body chemistry. If you do become physically or mentally distressed, in one way or another, make sure that you eat correctly. Go on Food Plan III at the end of the book so that you will not be adding more stress to your body with the food that you eat.

All distress changes the body chemistry in the same way, whether the distress comes from foods your body cannot utilize, physical or mental distress, or any combination of these. If you have legal problems, business problems, or personal problems, try to make sure you eat well, get some exercise, and do whatever you need to do to take the mental stress off your body.

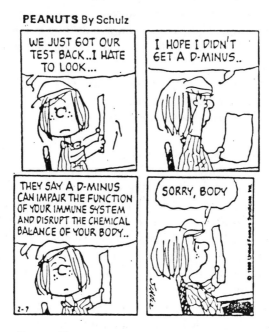

Reprinted by permission of UFS, Inc.

It is easier to deal with mental stress than physical stress. Today, there are many methods of stress reduction: individual and group therapy, exercise, meditation, journal writing, biofeedback, deep breathing, yoga, and body work such as massage, rolfing, and Heller work. Many books and tapes are available for mental, psychological, and spiritual growth. Each person must find the best method for him or herself.

I can remember when I spent much of each day depressed, angry, or resentful toward other people. I also had allergies, arthritis, headaches, yeast infections, and continual recurrences of boils and canker sores. By age forty, I had lost one inch off of my height. Boy, was I a candidate for osteoporosis! Finally, I changed my lifestyle. I started eating healthy foods and removed the junk from my diet.

Most importantly, I began psychotherapy. I spent three years with a psychoanalyst and also spent time in various group therapies. A one week workshop with Elizabeth Kübler-Ross and her book *Death and Dying* changed my attitude toward life and death. *The Course in Miracles* gave me strength.

It was important to get my body and my mind working together—working for, not against me. For many of us, our minds keep our bodies from getting well. The mind says, "I want an ice cream cone." The body says, "I don't need that." In my case, body work helped bring my body and mind closer. I experienced the deep muscular and organ massage provided by rolfing. Through Heller work, my body was brought back into its proper alignment. Jack Rosenberg's book *Body, Self & Soul* gave me new insights into the body-mind connection. *Conversational Rape* by Pat Allen gave me a new slant on relationships. And the list goes on.

We have too many "yes . . . buts" in our lives. Change is evolutionary, not revolutionary. Once you get on with the process of understanding yourself, it is hard to stop. I constantly read new books in the psychological field. I attend lectures and seminars and listen to tapes. The process just goes on. Change takes time and is difficult. In our fast-paced lives, all we can really hang our hat on is change.

In order for our civilization to survive, we are going to have to make some changes. Once we stop evolving, we are in for problems. All of life is evolving. In this sense, life is survival of the fit—the most physically and mentally fit. Those who do not see that each of us is creating his or her own illness will not be as healthy, will not live as long, and will create future generations whose bodies will be weaker.

After spending too many years frustrated and angry, I know it is possible to wake up happy and go to sleep the same way. Until you do the same, don't stop searching for the right methods and answers for you. As Jack Rosenberg says, "Mental health is a series of pleasant days." How true that is.

Distress is the main cause of upset body chemistry, but there are other parts of our twentieth century lifestyle that create an imbalance in our bodies as well. There are things that each of us does to keep the homeostatic mechanisms from working properly, and, therefore, continue to keep our body out of balance.

Sugar

Sugar is one of the basic substances that can upset homeostasis. I don't even call it a food. It is a chemical our bodies cannot utilize or digest well. When I say sugar, I don't simply mean table sugar, but also raw sugar, brown sugar, turbinado sugar, glucose, maple syrup, honey, fructose, rice syrup, barley malt, corn syrup, dextrose, and dextrine as well.

These simple sugars get into the bloodstream very quickly after being swallowed. They need very little digestion, and they do not have to go all the way through the normal digestive path. Some simple sugar can be absorbed right under the tongue. It is the speed as well as the quantity that gets into the bloodstream and causes the upset. The more sugar consumed, the more upset the body chemistry can become.

Dr. Melvin Page was one of the first to prove that eating sugar changes the calcium/phosphorus ratio in the blood and, therefore, changes the whole body chemistry. A simple blood test before and after eating sugar showed that calcium and phosphorus change their relationship to each other, with the calcium usually going up and the phosphorus going down. Page continued to monitor the calcium/phosphorus ratio for as long as forty-eight hours after the ingestion of sugar. He found that some people would stay out of homeostasis for more than twenty-four hours after eating sugar.

Page was not the only one to find this relationship between sugar and the loss of homeostasis. Other researchers have found that not only an excess of calcium, but also magnesium is secreted into the urine after glucose ingestion. When an excess is excreted in this way, the chemical makeup is changed and the body chemistry is upset. In Czechoslovakia, researchers found that excessive amounts of sucrose disturbed the metabolism of all the minerals.

The Department of Nutritional Science at the University of Connecticut studied the blood samples of people before and after they ingested two grams of sucrose per kilogram of body weight. That would be equivalent to twenty-nine teaspoons of sugar for a person weighing 150 pounds. Sugar consumption increased the level of insulin in the blood and reduced the level of phosphorus. Urinary excretion of zinc and sodium was also increased as a result of this sugar ingestion. The researchers concluded that a high sugar intake inhibits calcium from the kidneys and increases their urinary excretion. It certainly upsets the body chemistry.

You can be putting the right amount of calcium into your body, but when eaten with sugar, that calcium will not absorb efficiently. Dr. J. B. Orr showed that rickets, a calcium deficiency generally found in children, could be induced by the use of sweetened condensed milk. He felt that this deficiency was caused by the "dilution" of the minerals in the original milk as a result of the sweetening.

Orr didn't understand that all minerals work in relation to each other, but he did understand that the calcium in this sweetened condensed milk could not be utilized by the body. He also found it fascinating that the dilution of the minerals in no way affected the caloric content of the milk, which stayed the same, sweetened or unsweetened.

Dr. Joseph Schneider goes on to say that, "The ills often laid at the doors of sucrose and other highly refined carbohydrates are more properly explainable on the grounds that they act as a dilutant of the necessary mineral content of the food." The information is out there. It is no secret.

The main abuser of sugar within the food industry is the soft drink industry. Americans drink an average of 380 sugared soft drinks a year per person. Each of those soft drinks has approximately ten teaspoons of sugar. Therefore, in soft drinks alone we consume almost eleven teaspoons of sugar per day per person.

You might be surprised to know how many other food items have sugar in them. Start reading labels; you'll find sugar listed on the labels of bacon, pastrami, packaged pizza, salt, hot dogs, bologna, NutraSweet, non-dairy creamers, canned vegetables, and breads, to name just a few. Sugar is a cheap filler at thirty-five cents a pound, but that's not the only reason it is so widely used. Manufacturers know that the sweetness is addicting and keeps us coming back for more. They want us to get hooked on their products and buy more. Check the sugar content of the different foods found in Table 3.1. You might be surprised.

There's no doubt about it: sugar tastes good! If I had my choice today, I'd rather sit down to a pound of chocolate than my vegetables, but I don't because I know what it does to my body.

Dairy Products

The American Dairy Industry, through its advertising, leads us to believe that milk is beneficial for everyone. Statistics prove that this is not the case. Dairy products contain a sugar called lactose. When a person has a negative reaction to milk or other dairy products, one of the most common reasons is that the person does not have enough lactase (an enzyme) to digest the lactose. Lactose intolerance is common in most ethnic groups, occurring in 70 percent of Black Americans and over 70 percent of Jews, Arabs, Greeks, Japanese, Eskimos,

Table 3.1   The Sour Facts About Sugar

Product	Amount	Sugar Content (teaspoons)
BEVERAGES		
Gatorade	8 ounces	3.3
Ovaltine Malt Flavoring	4–5 teaspoons	4.3
Nestea Iced Tea, presweetened	8 ounces	5.7
Nestle's Hot Cocoa Mix	1 ounce	5.8
Kool-Aid, presweetened	8 ounces	6.0
Carnation Chocolate Slender	10 ounces	6.3
Hawaiian Punch	8 ounces	6.5
Hi-C Grape Drink	8 ounces	7.3
Tang	8 ounces	7.6
Canada Dry Ginger Ale	12 ounces	8.0
Canada Dry Tonic Water	12 ounces	8.4
Coca Cola	12 ounces	9.8
Pepsi Cola	12 ounces	10.0
Mountain Dew	12 ounces	11.0
Shasta Orange Soda	12 ounces	11.8
BREAKFAST CEREALS		
Lucky Charms	1 ounce	2.8
Cocoa Puffs	1 ounce	2.8
Sugar Frosted Flakes	1 ounce	2.8
Sugar Corn Pops	1 ounce	3.0
Cap'n Crunch	1 ounce	3.0
Froot Loops	1 ounce	3.3
Apple Jacks	1 ounce	3.5
Quaker Instant Oatmeal, Maple and Brown Sugar	1.5 ounces	3.5
Quaker Instant Oatmeal, Cinnamon and Spice	1.5 ounces	4.3
CAKES		
Cupcakes with icing	2¹/₂ inches in diameter	3.2
Gingerbread, no icing	2.3 ounces	4.1
Hostess Twinkie	1	4.8
Angel food cake, no icing	3.2 ounces	6.8
Sara Lee Chocolate Cake	3.2 ounces	7.9
Black forest cake	3.2 ounces	10.0
Sponge cake with icing	3.2 ounces	10.7

Table 3.1—*Continued*

Product	Amount	Sugar Content (teaspoons)
CANDY		
M&Ms, peanut	14	3.0
M&Ms, plain	31	3.5
Reese's Peanut Butter Cup	1.6 ounces	4.8
Marshmallows	4 large	5.3
Jelly beans	10	6.6
CANDY BARS		
Hershey's Milk Chocolate with Almonds	1 ounce	3.2
Nestle's Crunch	1 ounce	3.2
Hershey's Milk Chocolate	1 ounce	3.4
Milky Way	1 ounce	3.9
DAIRY PRODUCTS		
Heinz Custard Pudding (baby food)	4.5 ounces	3.9
Dannon low-fat yogurt, flavored	1 cup	4.2
Vanilla ice milk	1 cup	5.4
Dannon frozen yogurt, vanilla	1 cup	5.6
Vanilla ice cream	1 cup	5.8
Dannon low-fat yogurt, with fruit	1 cup	6.0
Dannon frozen yogurt, with fruit	1 cup	7.4
Thick shake	11 ounces	9.6
Ice cream sandwich	1 cup	19.0
FRUITS AND VEGETABLES (canned)		
Cream-style corn	1/2 cup	1.5
Peaches in light syrup	1/2 cup	2.3
Pineapple in heavy syrup	1/2 cup	3.0
Sweet potatoes in syrup	1/2 cup	3.1
Pears in heavy syrup	1/2 cup	3.6
Beets with Harvard sauce	1/2 cup	3.8

Product	Amount	Sugar Content (teaspoons)
Peaches in heavy syrup	1/2 cup	4.3
OTHER DESSERTS AND SNACKS		
Jelly doughnut	1.8 ounces	1.7
Glazed doughnut	1.5 ounces	1.8
Heinz Dutch Apple Desert (baby food)	4.5 ounces	2.2
Eclair with icing	3.5 ounces	2.8
Blueberry or Cherry Pop-Tart	1.8 ounces	3.3
Chocolate pudding from mix	1/2 cup	4.1
Jello	1/2 cup	4.2
Hunts Snack Pack, vanilla	4.25 ounces	4.4
Popsicle	1	4.5
Frosted Chocolate Fudge Pop-Tart	1.8 ounces	4.5
Sherbet	1/2 cup	6.7
Caramel apple	1	7.6
PIES		
Pumpkin	4.6 ounces	3.6
Cherry	4.6 ounces	4.4
Peach	4.6 ounces	4.5
Apple	4.6 ounces	4.9
Lemon meringue	4.6 ounces	7.8
Pecan	4.6 ounces	12.0

Reprinted from CSPI's SugarScoreboard, available from the Center for Science in the Public Interest, 1875 Connecticut Ave., NW, Suite 300, Washington, D.C. 20009-5728 for $4.95, copyright 1985.

Indians, Africans, and Asians. Statistics show that in the United States, 50 percent of all people tested for food allergies have reactions to dairy products. Out of all the allergic substances, milk and milk products head the list.

When we eat food that we are allergic to, we upset our body chemistries and the food is not absorbed well. So, for those with a lactose intolerance, eating and drinking milk products can actually lead to osteoporosis.

I am allergic to milk and milk products. When I was in college, I had a calcium deposit the size of a grapefruit removed from my chest. I do not eat any dairy products and, though I may be over fifty years of age, I have no osteoporosis. I test my urine for homeostasis regularly (order form found on back page), and I eat according to the food plan outlined in Chapter 5 of this book. I make sure I include fish, dark green vegetables, red and orange vegetables, soy products, and small amounts of seeds and nuts in my diet.

If dairy products seem right for you, then by all means eat and drink them. However, if they cause symptoms such as cramping, gas, bloating, falling asleep after eating them, fatigue, headaches, or constipation, then I suggest you look for other sources of calcium in your diet. Stop upsetting your body chemistry. Any of the diets described in the back of the book will give you enough absorbable calcium.

In Asia and Africa diets are low in calcium. These native diets do not include milk products—no milk, cheese, yogurt, cottage cheese, or ice cream. The average calcium intake is somewhere between 300–500 milligrams of calcium per day, however, osteoporosis is virtually unknown in these civilizations where people eat their native foods. These people get their calcium from soy, dark green vegetables, carrots, fish, seeds, and nuts. In Europe and North American, where the consumption of calcium is much greater (800–1,000 milligrams of calcium per day), osteoporosis is becoming an epidemic.

Table 3.2 lists some common dairy products and their calcium contents, but remember, it is not enough to simply put the correct number of milligrams of calcium into your mouth. This will not necessarily produce a desirable effect. For example, having a twelve-ounce milkshake for lunch, which has 600 milligrams of calcium, and fruit yogurt for dinner, which has 600 milligrams of calcium, would seem like plenty of calcium for the day, right? Wrong. The sugar in the milkshake (approximately five teaspoons) and in the fruit yogurt (seven teaspoons) so upsets the body chemistry that the calcium you have eaten cannot all be absorbed. Not only are you absorbing

Table 3.2   Dairy Products and Calcium

Product	Amount	Calcium Content (milligrams)
Half-and-half	1 tablespoon	16
Cottage cheese	1/2 cup	140
Camembert	1 ounce	150
Bleu cheese	1 ounce	150
Mozzarella cheese	1 ounce	160
Cheddar cheese	1 ounce	200
Provolone cheese	1 ounce	210
Ricotta cheese (whole milk)	1/2 cup	216
Swiss cheese	1 ounce	270
Milk (whole)	8 ounces	290
Buttermilk	8 ounces	290
Milk (low-fat)	8 ounces	310
Yogurt, plain (low-fat)	8 ounces	400

Based upon information from *The Calcium Bible* by Hausman, Patricia, M.S. New York: Warner Books, 1985.

less of the calcium in the sugary milk products, but the other minerals and nutrients are also less available to your body. Sugar, though not the only thing that pulls calcium from the bones, is certainly one of the worst offenders.

So listen to your body and test it. If your body is happy with dairy products, then use them. If not, don't. Just don't fool yourself into believing that you are getting usable calcium in milkshakes, ice cream cones, cheesecake, and fruit yogurt.

Salt

You are, undoubtedly, aware that too much salt is unhealthy. It can raise your blood pressure and in so doing increase your risk of hypertension, kidney disease, and heart and vascular disease. But another health hazard of salt is the risk of losing large amounts of calcium in the urine. This loss is directly related to the quantity of table salt in the diet, not the salt found in fruits and vegetables. The more sodium chloride (table salt) you ingest, the more sodium and calcium you excrete.

It is difficult to say how much salt is too much in terms of its effect on calcium balance. One study showed that when sodium intake was limited to 200 milligrams per day, there was no change in the amount of calcium excreted. Two thousand milligrams a day, however, led to a significant increase of calcium in the urine.

Another researcher, Ailsa Goulding, Ph.D., of the University of Otago in New Zealand, found that animals given salt supplements lost more calcium and phosphorus in their urine and had less of these minerals in their skeletons than those animals not receiving salt. In another study, Dr. Goulding found that adding a teaspoon of table salt daily to the diet of young women increased the amount of calcium lost—enough to decrease bone mass by an estimated 1.5 percent per year. Again, don't worry about the natural salt found in fruits and vegetables. The culprit is table salt, the same salt used in processed foods. Table 3.3 shows the surprisingly high content of sodium found in common processed foods.

There are other forms of sodium than those found in table salt. Actually, few of us realize how much sodium we dose ourselves with daily. Sodium nitrate is used to preserve many processed foods. Scientists have discovered that sodium nitrate can cause cancerous tumors if ingested over a period of years. Sodium nitrate is found in hot dogs, bacon, cold cuts, and some canned fish. Did you realize it is possible to ingest these dangerous compounds while cooking? When you cook bacon, high levels of sodium nitrate can actually be inhaled into your body, and the levels can be as high as four times the amount obtained by just eating the bacon!

Another way to obtain sodium is through monosodium glutamate, commonly known as MSG. It is commonly found

Table 3.3   Sodium Content of Common Processed Foods

Product	Amount	Sodium Content (milligrams)
BEVERAGES		
Soft drinks, regular	8 oz.	11
Soft drinks, diet	8 oz.	29
Club soda	8 oz.	56
Tomato juice	6 oz.	659
Vegetable juice	6 oz.	659
BREADS AND CRACKERS		
Biscuit mix, with milk	1 biscuit	272
Bread, white	1 slice	114
Bread, whole wheat	1 slice	132
Roll, hard	1 roll	313
CEREALS (non sugar-coated)		
Bran flakes (40 percent)	1 oz. (2/3 cup)	265
Corn flakes	1 oz. (1 cup)	350
Wheat flakes	1 oz. (1 cup)	370
CONDIMENTS, DRESSINGS, and SEASONINGS		
Catsup	1 tablespoon	156
Salad dressing, French	1 tablespoon	214
Salt, table	1 teaspoon	2,325
Soy sauce	1 tablespoon	1,029
DAIRY PRODUCTS, EGGS, and MARGARINE		
Cheese, American	1 slice	406
Cheese, cheddar	1 oz.	176
Cheese, cottage	1/2 cup	457
Cheese, Parmesan (grated)	1 oz.	528
Milk, buttermilk	8 oz.	257
Milk, low-fat (2 percent)	8 oz.	122
FISH and SEAFOOD (canned)		
Crabmeat, drained	4 oz.	1,250
Sardines, drained	3.25 oz.	598
Tuna (in oil), drained	3.25 oz.	328
MEAT and POULTRY		
Bacon	2 slices (1/2 oz.)	274
Bologna	1 slice	224

Table 3.3—*Continued*

Product	Amount	Sodium Content (milligrams)
Beef, corned	2 slices (3 oz.)	802
Frankfurter, all meat	1	639
Ham, cured lean	2 slices (4 oz.)	1,494
Liverwurst (Braunschweiger)	1 slice	324
Sausage, pork	1 patty (2 oz.)	259
PASTA		
Macaroni and cheese	1 cup	1,086
Spaghetti with tomato sauce and cheese	1 cup	955
SOUPS (commercial varieties)		
Beef broth	1 cup	1,152
Chicken, cream of (with milk	1 cup	1,054
Chicken noodle	1 cup	1,107
Onion	1 cup	1,051
Tomato	1 cup	872
CANNED/BOTTLED FOODS		
Asparagus	4 spears	298
Beans, baked (with pork and tomato sauce)	1/2 cup	319
Beans, green	1/2 cup	319
Beans, lima	1/2 cup	228
Beets	1/2 cup	240
Corn, creamed	1/2 cup	336
Peas, green	1/2 cup	247
Pickles, dill	1 spear	232
Sauerkraut	1/2 cup	777
Spinach	1/2 cup	455
SNACKS		
Corn chips	1 oz.	231
Cashews, dry-roasted and salted	4 tablespoons (1 oz.)	150
Potato chips	14 chips (1 oz.)	285
Pretzels, regular twist	5 pretzels (1/2 oz.)	505

Based upon information from *Killer Salt* by Whittlesey, Marietta. New York: Avon Books, 1978.

in Chinese food, as well as canned, frozen, and packaged foods. MSG is used to enhance flavor. It can be purchased by the shaker, and although it tastes less salty than table salt, it has three times the sodium content. So watch out for MSG!

Caffeine

Caffeine, another substance that causes an excess of calcium to be secreted into the urine, is becoming a larger and larger part of our diets. It is found in coffee, tea, soft drinks, and chocolate. Caffeine is even found in many prescription and non-prescription medications; it is contained in some cold medicines, headache relievers, and allergy remedies, to name just a few. According to the Food and Drug Administration, more than 1,000 over-the-counter drugs show caffeine as a listed ingredient. The statistics found in Table 3.4, 3.5, and 3.6 will give you an idea of just how much caffeine we ingest each day.

What effect does all of this caffeine have on our body chemistries? One study showed that whenever a person drinks three cups of caffeinated coffee, forty-five milligrams of calcium is secreted into the urine. Sodium and potassium are also secreted. As we have seen, when one mineral becomes deficient due to excess secretion in the urine, all of the other minerals become upset and can become excess and toxic, or deficient.

Twelve healthy young women who habitually consumed an average of 300 milligrams of caffeine per day (five cups of coffee) were studied for the effects of caffeine on mineral excretion. After an overnight fast, all the subjects were given decaffeinated coffee or tea. Six of the subjects unknowingly took the decaffeinated beverage with 300 milligrams of caffeine added. During the three hours following, both groups

Table 3.4   Caffeine Content of Foods and Beverages

Product	Caffeine (average milligrams)
COFFEE (5 ounces)	
Brewed, drip method	80
Instant	65
Decaffeinated, brewed	3
Decaffeinated, instant	2
TEA (5 ounces)	
Brewed, major U.S. brands	40
Brewed, imported brands	60
Instant	30
Iced (12 ounces), brewed	70
COCOA (5 ounces)	4
CHOCOLATE MILK (8 ounces)	5
MILK CHOCOLATE (1 ounce)	5
DARK CHOCOLATE, semi-sweet (1 ounce)	6
BAKER'S CHOCOLATE (1 ounce)	26
CHOCOLATE-FLAVORED SYRUP (1 ounce)	4

SOURCE: FDA, Food Additive Chemistry Evaluation Branch, based on evaluations of existing literature on caffeine levels.

were checked for excess minerals in their urine. The group that took the decaffeinated coffee without added caffeine had no excess minerals. The group that took the beverage with the added caffeine, had a 42 percent increase in magnesium in their urine and the sodium and calcium was increased by 142 percent.

In addition, the total urinary output was 30 percent greater after drinking the caffeinated coffee. Caffeine is a natural diuretic. It makes you secrete more urine. Caffeine caused a total excess magnesium loss of 4.9 milligrams,

Table 3.5 Caffeine Content of Soft Drinks

Product	Caffeine (mgs per 12-ounce serving)
CARBONATED	
cherry coke, Coca-Cola	46
cherry cola Slice	48
cherry RC	36
Coca-Cola	46
Coca-Cola Classic	46
cola	37
cola, RC	36
Mello Yello	52
Mr. Pibb	40
Mountain Dew	54
pepper-type soda	37
Pepsi Cola	38
CARBONATED, LOW CALORIE	
diet cherry coke, Coca-Cola	46
diet cherry cola Slice	48
diet coke, Coca-Cola	46
diet cola, aspartame sweetened	50
diet Pepsi	36
diet RC	48
Pepsi Light	36
Tab	46

SOURCE: Bowes and Church, *Food Values of Portions Commonly Used*, 15th ed., rev. Jean A. T. Pennington (Philadelphia: J. B. Lippincott Company, 1989).

which would more than offset the magnesium contained in the coffee. The authors of the study concluded that a high level of caffeine consumption may increase the risk of calcium deficiency, as well as the deficiency of other vital nutrients.

In a group of post-menopausal women with reduced amounts of bone, it was found that 31 percent of the women drank four or more cups of coffee every day. In a group of women with normal bones, only 3 percent drank that amount of coffee. We don't know how much sugar these people consumed in their diets, per day, along with the four cups of cof-

Table 3.6 Caffeine Content of Drugs

Product	Caffeine (mgs per tablet)
PRESCRIPTION DRUGS	
Cafergot (for migraine headaches)	100
Darvon Compound (pain reliever)	32.4
Fiorinal (for tension headaches)	40
Soma Compound (pain reliever, muscle relaxant)	32
WEIGHT-CONTROL AIDS (non-prescription)	
Appedrine, Maximum-Strength	100
Codexin	200
Dex-A-Diet II	200
Dexatrim, Extra-Strength	200
Diatac Capsules	200
Prolamine	140
ALERTNESS TABLETS (non-prescription)	
No Doz	100
Vivarin	200
HEADACHE/PAIN RELIEVERS (non-prescription)	
Anacin, Maximum-Strength	32
Dristan	16
Empirin	32
Excedrin	65
Midol	32.4
DIURETICS (non-prescription)	
Aqua-Ban	100
Aqua-Ban Plus, Maximum-Strength	200
Permathene H2 Off	200
COLD/ALLERGY REMEDIES (non-prescription)	
Coryban-D capsules	30
Dristan decongestant tablets	16.2
Dristan A-F decongestant tablets	16.2
Duradyne-Forte	30
Triaminicin tablets	30

SOURCE: Food and Drug Administration, National Center for Drug and Biologics.

fee, but that too would play a role in the calcium loss. Of course, how they dealt with stress could also have been a factor.

A study conducted at Washington State University suggests that both caffeine and sugar intake have a negative effect on calcium balance, and that the calcium loss may be greatest when these two dietary factors are consumed together. In this study, teen-agers, from thirteen to eighteen years of age, consumed caffeine-free, sugar-free soft drinks with either sugar, caffeine, or sugar and caffeine added. Urine was collected after each study and tested for calcium excretion values. Calcium loss increased following ingestion of either sugar or caffeine, but was greatest when the two were consumed together. Caffeine alone caused both an increased concentration of calcium in the urine and an increased urine volume. Sugar alone did not increase urine volume, but substantially increased urinary calcium concentration. Year after year of abuse like this can bring on osteoporosis quicker than you think!

Tobacco

A number of apparent links have been found between smoking and osteoporosis. Women who smoke reach menopause an average of five years earlier than non-smokers. Even passive exposure to secondary cigarette smoke has been shown to cause an earlier average age of menopause. Cigarette smoking has been shown to stop estrogen activity, and anything that stops estrogen from functioning is likely to cause osteoporosis.

Information from the Argonne National Laboratory indicates that cadmium (a heavy metal) might be one of the problems for cigarette smokers. Cadmium is found in cigarette smoke and can cause extensive bone loss. Animal studies have shown that even extremely low levels of cadmium (similar to those in women who smoke) can result in a 30 percent loss of bone calcium.

The sooner you stop smoking, the more likely you are to have stronger bones, not to mention avoiding the other problems associated with tobacco, such as lung cancer, cardiovascular disease, and emphysema. Each of the current smokers in the United States will, on the average, save the government about $35,000 in social security payments by dying sooner than non-smokers. Do you really want to do the government that much of a favor?

Alcohol

The relationship between bone disease and alcohol abuse is well established. A large percentage of individuals whose drinking habits have caused them to seek medical help can be diagnosed, with routine x-rays, as having osteoporosis. Researchers at a Veterans Administration Hospital in Illinois found extensive bone loss in those patients who were chronic alcoholics.

Tests of alcoholics show that there are less minerals in their bones, and even young alcoholics show evidence of decreased bone mass. The degree to which osteoporosis is present in the overall drinking population remains uncertain, but most osteoporosis in middle-aged men can be attributed to alcohol abuse.

It is not only alcohol abuse that can cause osteoporosis. The November 1989 issue of *Longevity* reports on a study done at the University of California—San Diego School of Medicine, La Jolla. This study reports that as little as two drinks in a day could cut the benefits of calcium in one's diet.

More than two glasses of wine, hard liquor, or beer in a day, will prevent the body from properly absorbing calcium and other important minerals.

Alcohol's effect on the body chemistry is a chain reaction. Not only does excess use of alcohol cause a decrease in the phosphorus level of the blood, but the drinker eats less and obtains very little phosphorus from food. In addition, because the minerals are not in the right relationship and enzymes are impaired, the food that is eaten does not digest well. Indigestion can be a problem. Antacids are then used, and the phosphorus is depleted even more. The only way out of this vicious cycle is to stop the excess use of alcohol.

Overcooked Foods

Overcooking food is another way to cause metabolic overload and upset body chemistry. All foods are made up of carbon, nitrogen, oxygen, and hydrogen in various chemical configurations. Our enzymes have evolved since the days of the caveman to digest foods in certain configurations. But when food is cooked at a high temperature, it passes what we call the *heat labile point*, which means that it changes its chemical configuration. Our enzymes don't know what to do with this overcooked food. We do not have evolutionary enzymes to digest it efficiently.

Since our enzymes cannot digest overcooked food very well, some of it does not digest at all. It sits partially digested in the gut and starts to putrify, or rot. This food putrification irritates the lining of the gastro-intestinal tract. The cells widen and the undigested food gets into the bloodstream where it can cause problems.

A study was done to find out how well different forms of calcium were absorbed. Pasteurized whole milk, dried whole milk, and homogenized whole milk were tested. It was found that the calcium in the dried milk preparation was definitely less well utilized. Why? Dried milk is prepared by pouring milk over stainless steel rolling drums that have been heated to a very high temperature. As the milk hits the drums, it loses its moisture. Small flakes drop off the drum and become dried milk. This is definitely overcooking.

In another study, researchers Barbara Schneeman and George Dunaif at the University of California, Davis, examined the browning reaction in food and how this usually produced better taste, but less efficient digestibility. For four weeks, they fed laboratory rats nonfat milk as their only source of protein. One group of rats received unheated milk. A second group ingested milk heated to a light brown at 121° C. The third group was given milk cooked to a cocoa brown.

Rats given the unheated milk thrived. They grew and gained wight. Rats given the light-brown milk failed to gain weight. Rats given the cocoa-brown milk took in less food and lost weight. The researchers discovered that browned proteins stay longer in the stomach, indicating poor digestibility and poor absorption. This research indicates that drinking milk in its raw form is the best.

Fried foods are particularly dangerous. When a food is fried and becomes brown, the chemical configuration of the food changes and our enzymes are less capable of digesting it. This food gets into the bloodstream, undigested. The fat used to fry the food can clog the arteries as well as upset the body chemistry.

When foods are deep fried—whether they be potatoes, shrimp, carrots, or chicken—a vat of oil is heated to a very high temperature, far above the heat labile point. Then food is dropped into this vat and fried. Afterwards, the vat of oil is cooled down. This same vat is usually heated up again to cook more food. The fat used can quickly become rancid. We do not have enzymes to digest rancid fats, and the body chemistry becomes upset once again.

The best methods for cooking food are steaming and baking. Food should be cooked at low temperatures for short periods of time. Eat as much raw food as you possibly can. Check the food plans in Chapter 5 for more information.

Protein

When the body's pH balance becomes acidic, calcium is pulled from the bones to buffer this acidic state, thereby weakening the bones. One of the main factors that causes this acidic state is excess protein.

Dr. Uriel S. Barzel, M.D., from Albert Einstein College of Medicine in New York, showed that the long-term ingestion of excess acid through protein digestion caused osteoporosis-like bone loss in rats. The bone loss developed as a response to the physiological stress imposed on the animal by the acid state.

Early research into high protein diets showed an increased calcium absorption, but the magnitude of this increase did not offset the increased urinary calcium loss. Other studies show that when you eat a high protein diet, your phosphorus level drops; therefore, all that excess calcium, which can no longer work in relation to the phosphorus, can become toxic and/or be excreted into the urine.

Whenever you do something to upset your body chemistry, such as eating too much protein, excess calcium can be excreted into the urine. The Arctic Eskimos, whose main diet is fish, have a far greater bone loss than other people in the same region eating a diet with less protein.

When the body is giving off excess calcium in the urine, the body is out of homeostasis and in for trouble. Ninety-five grams of protein per day will cause a daily calcium loss of twenty-six milligrams. This loss may be due to the high concentration of acid ash, which is the end product of meat digestion and which the body tries to neutralize by dissolving calcium and phosphorus from the bones.

Amino acids, a breakdown product of protein metabolism, have also been found to cause excess calcium secretion. Researchers found that the percentage of calcium in the urine increased as the amino acids increased. They also discovered that the phosphorus increased in the diet as the protein increased. The effect of excessive phosphorus in the gut was said to be the most important factor in relating why there was excess calcium in the urine. These researchers understood that the excess phosphorus in the diet caused extra calcium to be excreted, but they never saw the whole picture, they didn't realize that all minerals (not just calcium and phosphorus) work in relation to each other.

Each person is able to handle a different amount of protein. It depends on how depleted the buffer systems are. Keep the information found in Table 3.7 in mind when deciding how much protein you are eating or can eat. You might be surprised at how high in protein certain foods are, and how little protein others contain.

There is a test that can help you discover the amount of protein you can handle. Using the kit that can be ordered from the back page of this book, first test the pH of your saliva. Next, eat an eight-ounce serving of broiled or baked beef, chicken, fish, or pork at one sitting. Make sure not to eat anything else. Test your saliva again. If your saliva becomes acidic, you have exhausted your buffer system and you are not only acidic, but can be losing calcium from your bones as well.

I would like to say a few things about vegetarianism. If you are a vegetarian, our program will suit you fine. On any one of the food plans, it is possible to combine beans and grains to get complete protein. Many meat eaters in our society are "protein logged" today—bacon and eggs for breakfast, hamburgers for lunch, and meat and potatoes for dinner. That's too much protein, and we have learned that too

Table 3.7   Protein Content of Common Foods

Product	Amount	Protein (grams)
DAIRY and EGGS		
Cottage cheese (creamed)	¹/₂ cup	15.6
Milk	1 cup	8.0
Cheddar cheese	1 ounce	7.1
Egg	1 medium	6.5
MEAT AND FISH		
Tuna, canned and drained	4 ounces	31.0
Chicken	4 ounces, cooked	24.5
Hamburger	4 ounces, cooked	32.0
Sirloin steak	4 ounces, cooked	31.0
GRAINS		
Whole wheat flour	¹/₂ cup	7.5
Spaghetti	1 cup, cooked	5.0
Cornmeal	¹/₂ cup	7.8
Rice, brown	1 cup, cooked	5.0
Rice, white	1 cup, cooked	4.0
LEGUMES		
Soybeans	¹/₂ cup, cooked	9.8
Peanut butter	1 ounce	7.9
Lima beans	¹/₂ cup, cooked	7.0
Cashews	1 ounce	4.8

SOURCE: Watt, Bernice K., and Merrill, Annabel. "Composition of Foods." *Agricultural Handbook*, no. 8 (1975). U.S. Department of Agriculture, Washington, D.C.

much protein can cause osteoporosis. If you are a vegetarian, you probably do not eat too much protein, unless you are obsessed with cheese and eggs.

Vegetarians can have problems with clogged arteries because many vegetarians still eat sugar. The body manufactures its own cholesterol, even if one does not eat it. Eating sugar can upset the body chemistry, which can make some of the calcium non-functioning or toxic. This toxic calcium can cling to the cholesterol, causing the arteries to harden. Many vegetarians have eliminated sugar from their diets, which is certainly a good idea.

A meat eater should remember to boil, poach, steam, or bake chicken, fish, beef, and eggs. Do not fry, sauté, or barbecue. Remember to eat small portions.

This book is about osteoporosis, not hardened arteries, but any way we upset our body chemistry can cause clogged arteries in some and osteoporosis in others. Some unfortunates can get both.

Phosphorus

Americans have doubled their average daily intake of phosphorus over the past forty years, from less than 800 milligrams to over 1,400 milligrams. During the same period of time, the average daily intake of other essential minerals such as calcium and magnesium have declined, leaving the dietary calcium to phosphorus ratio far short of the optimum 2.5 to 1.

Those who drink soft drinks consume even more phosphorus. Soft drinks—regular, sugar-free and/or caffeine-free—contain phosphoric acid. This phosphoric acid is a form of phosphorus, and excess phosphorus can upset the delicate mineral balance and cause a calcium deficiency.

It would seem logical to simply add extra calcium to the diet to bring the ratio back to normal. But in fact, as both calcium and phosphorus are increased, a strange thing happens. Phosphorus will be absorbed efficiently even at very high intakes, but the efficiency of calcium absorption at high intakes decreases sharply. As the level of both elements is increased proportionally, the ratio of absorbed calcium to phosphorus shifts in favor of the latter, and the minerals are upset all over again.

When a person upsets his or her body chemistry by consuming more phosphorus than the body can handle, an excess of phosphorus gets into the bloodstream. The calcium that is there forms an insoluble complex with the phosphorus. This causes less functioning calcium in the blood, so the parathyroid is stimulated to secrete its hormone, which can pull calcium out of the bones.

A delicate balance must be maintained between the calcium and the phosphorus. If too much calcium is consumed, it will become toxic. If too much phosphorus is consumed and gets into the bloodstream, there will not be enough calcium in the blood to balance the phosphorus, so more calcium is pulled from the bones. Not only can phosphorus bind calcium in the intestines and make it unavailable, but it can also bind other essential trace minerals such as magnesium, manganese, zinc, and copper.

There is a widespread use of phosphorus additives in the food industry today. These substances consist mainly of such salts as orthophosphates, pyrophosphates, and polysulphates. These are used as chelators, emulsifying agents, and binders. Start reading your labels to find out how much phosphorus you are getting from non-food sources. You will be amazed.

There is one study of interest that shows what phosphate additives can do. One group of adults, the control group, was fed a normal diet consisting of 700 milligrams of calcium, 95 grams of protein and 2,200 calories. This diet included fresh meat, yeast bread, and natural cheese. A second group of adults was fed the same normal diet, but with a few crucial changes. Processed meat was substituted for the fresh meat, refrigerator rolls for the yeast rolls, and processed cheese for the natural.

This resulted in an increase in phosphorus intake of 1.1 grams per day. There was a rise in serum phosphate, a decrease in serum calcium, a decrease in urinary calcium, and indications of parathyroid stimulation, meaning that calcium was probably pulled from the bone.

The contribution of food additives to the total intake of phosphorus is not well documented, but it could represent a large source of phosphorus in our food supply. The use of food additives has grave implications for calcium and bone metabolism.

Calcium Supplements

Taking extra calcium in the form of supplements may seem the obvious way to combat a calcium deficiency. The sale of calcium supplements has increased dramatically since 1983, as middle-aged women seek to prevent or stop bone loss due to osteoporosis. However, I believe that studies have failed to support the hypothesis that large amounts of calcium are associated with increased bone density or a decreased incidence of fracture. Instead, they may actually help cause osteoporosis by upsetting the mineral relationships and therefore the body chemistry.

Some researchers believe that the calcium you take as an adult has little to do with whether you will get osteoporosis or not. Dr. B. Lawrence Riggs of the Mayo Clinic studied 107 women who were twenty-three to eight-eight years old. They were studied for over four years. During that time, Riggs and his associates repeatedly measured their bone density.

The women consumed from 269 to 2,000 milligrams of calcium a day, and the daily intake of calcium was steady for each woman throughout the study period. The results showed that there was no correlation at all between calcium intake and bone loss, not even a trend. Even when Riggs took into account age, menopause status, and serum estrogen levels, there was no correlation.

Furthermore, Riggs found that the women in the upper quartile of calcium intake (those consuming more than 1,400 milligrams of calcium each day) had the same amount of bone loss as those in the lower quartile (those consuming less than 500 milligrams a day).

Dr. Richard Mazess, of the University of Wisconsin, believes that there is an abundance of data showing that calcium intake in a population is unrelated to bone density. He points to quite a few population studies, including those done in the United States, the Netherlands, and Switzerland, which show that those who consumed the most calcium had no denser bones than those who consumed the least, taking into consideration body size and ethnic group.

Patients with severe osteoporosis were given massive doses of calcium and they went into a positive calcium balance. Most researchers feel that when you are in a positive calcium balance your body is absorbing enough calcium. When these patients had radiographic studies, there were no positive changes in the osteoporotic process. Where did all the calcium go? Probably into the soft tissue, where is does not belong.

Calcium supplements, therefore, do very little good, and they can do a great deal of harm. Supplements can have an adverse effect on the body's mineral relationships. One of the potential dangers in taking calcium supplements lies in the fact that excess calcium can be redistributed to deposit in soft tissues, causing arthritis, arteriosclerosis, kidney stones, and other problems.

Research from Tufts University on twenty-four healthy post-menopausal women showed that when 500 milligrams of elemental calcium, in the form of calcium carbonate, was added to the meal, iron retention was decreased to 45 percent in the control group that took no extra calcium with the meal. Many women sit on the border of an iron deficiency much of their lives. Women need to absorb and metabolize all of the iron they consume.

Fatigue is a common symptom of iron deficiency. Blood tests showing a low-normal iron and a low-normal red blood cell count are prevalent in many women. I believe that if those researchers had studied other minerals, they would have found some of those deficient also, because all minerals work in relation to one another. It has been suggested that calcium supplements should be taken with meals to insure better absorption, but this practice may actually decrease iron absorption.

Other studies show that taking excess calcium can deplete the magnesium in the body, just as taking excess magnesium can deplete the body's supply of calcium. A patient was admitted to a hospital complaining of malaise (a fatigued, run-down feeling) and stomach discomfort. Blood examination showed a very elevated magnesium level and very little calcium. When questioned, the man revealed that he had ingested large amounts of magnesium carbonate, in the form of an antacid, in an attempt to relieve his "indigestion."

Even though you may be getting sufficient quantities of calcium, if you take too much of another mineral, the calcium can become depleted. The opposite also holds true. If you take excess quantities of calcium, you can deplete other minerals in your body.

It is probably a good idea to take a vitamin and mineral supplement, but in a form that contains no sugar, wheat, dairy, fillers, food coloring, or carnuba wax. A hypo-allergenic pill from a health food store should do the trick, but taking extra calcium is questionable.

As long as you are upsetting your body chemistry, it doesn't matter how many supplements you ingest. If you take these supplements while eating a donut, the donut will so upset the body chemistry that the vitamins and minerals contained in the supplement will not be absorbed well. In fact, they can become toxic. Once again, the answer does not lie in miracle pills or supplements, but in returning the body to homeostasis.

Over-the-Counter and Prescription Drugs

There's no doubt that drugs save lives. Many people would not be living today if they had not taken the proper drug at the proper time. For short-term use, the right drug can be vitally important. However, research is being done on the long-term use of drugs, and many distressing side effects have been discovered.

Aspirin

Aspirin has long been hailed as a wonder drug, but there is evidence that aspirin may increase the permeability of the stomach and intestinal lining. If a person has food allergies, the simultaneous consumption of aspirin will allow more of the allergy-producing food to be absorbed. When undigested food gets into the bloodstream, it upsets the body chemistry and can cause excess calcium to be secreted into the urine. Based on certain reports in the *British Medical Journal*, it is recommended that people who have even the mildest forms of allergies to food should avoid taking aspirin and the food within several hours of each other. Better yet, find out why the aspirin is needed. Deal with the problem. Then there will be no need to take the aspirin and the aspirin will not be a problem.

Antibiotics

All of the antibiotics I tested resulted in excess calcium being secreted in the urine as long as the person is taking the drug. Among antibiotics, tetracycline is a well-known cause of bone damage and growth failure. If you need antibiotics, take them, but make sure you need them. If you do take antibiotics, also take acidophilus, for antibiotics not only kill the harmful bacteria, but also the good. Acidophilus will help to increase the helpful bacteria.

Acidophilus can be obtained in most health food stores. If possible, get the strongest one available (the one with the most lactobacillae). Make sure you take it the entire time you are taking the antibiotics. Continue taking it even after finishing the antibiotics. Finish the bottle.

Antacids

It is well documented that antacids can impair phosphorus absorption in man. Something in the antacids seems to bond with the phosphorus and escort it out of the body. Phosphorus deficiency may result from long-term treatment with antacids that contain magnesium hydroxide and/or aluminum hydroxide. When the phosphorus becomes depleted in the blood and in the urine, it decreases the gastro-intestinal absorption of calcium, while the calcium is increased in the blood. There is also a loss of skeletal calcium and phosphorus.

In other words, antacids upset the body chemistry. When the calcium goes up in the bloodstream and the phosphorus drops, all of the minerals can become toxic and/or non-functioning.

Dr. Herta Spencer, whose field is mineral metabolism, studied a group of men who took small amounts of antacids—actually, much less than the amount often used by patients with peptic ulcers. The results showed a loss of calcium and phosphorus in the blood. Dr. Spencer believes the prolonged depletion could lead to osteomalacia, which can lead to osteoporosis.

Long-term use of antacids causes phosphorus to become non-absorbable in the intestine. This may be due to the aluminum found in many antacids. Aluminum combines with the phosphorus in the intestines and results in an increase in fecal phosphorus excretion and therefore an inhibition of intestinal absorption of phosphorus. This decrease in phosphorus absorption is associated with an increase of calcium in the urine.

Patients on prolonged use of antacids often complain of bone pain, osteomalacia, pseudo-fractures, muscle weakness, debility, anorexia, and malaise. Patients who receive antacids in the hospital and continue to take them for a prolonged period of time have shown severe bone pain and x-ray evidence of substantial bone loss several years after the use of antacids started.

Because the phosphorus has been depleted, antacids lower the functioning calcium level. Since the parathyroid gland regulates the calcium metabolism, it becomes activated, causing an increase in the absorption of aluminum from food and water. A lower calcium level seems to increase the absorption of aluminum. Read your labels. Many antacids contain aluminum.

It is amazing to realize how many people use these over-the-counter drugs and think they are doing a good thing for their bodies. In fact, the body needs acid in the stomach in order for calcium to be absorbed. Calcium is absorbed in the upper part of the small intestine, and acid is essential.

That's why the frequent use of antacids wreaks havoc on the bones. People take antacids to deplete stomach acid, but this just makes the calcium more difficult to absorb. Stomach acid production decreases with age, and this might be one of the reasons why the efficiency of calcium absorption declines with age.

The antacid Tums is often promoted as a calcium supplement, because it contains calcium carbonate. Each tablet contains less than 20 percent of elemental calcium. But calcium needs magnesium to keep it from becoming non-functioning calcium in the form of kidney stones or arthritic spurs. As we have learned, minerals work in relation to each other. As calcium and phosphorus are important to each other, so are calcium and magnesium. Unfortunately, Tums is not only an antacid, but it also does not contain the magnesium necessary for calcium absorption. Tums is not a good answer to osteoporosis. The key lies in keeping the minerals in the right relationship for calcium to digest, metabolize, and function.

Why do so many people take antacids? Next to aspirin, more people take antacids than any other over-the-counter drug. People think they need antacids because their stomachs are upset after they eat. Antacids do stop the pain, but there is a much easier way to stop the pain: figure out what is causing it and eliminate that cause. There are various reasons why you get stomach pains after you eat. Let me suggest a few of these.

Stomachaches and overeating go hand-in-hand. Eating too much can exhaust your enzyme system, resulting in undigested food, which causes stomach pain. Other common reasons for stomach discomfort are eating foods your body is allergic to, consuming alcohol with meals, and eating desserts. For some people, combining simple sugars (such as those found in alcoholic drinks and desserts) with the protein eaten at dinner can result in stomachaches. Other reasons can include eating when you are in distress or when you are sick and your body chemistry is upset. During this time, food will not digest as well. Starve a cold and starve a fever. Eat as little as possible when you are sick, but drink plenty of fluids.

These are the main reasons that people need to take antacids. Next time you get stomach pains after you eat, try to figure out what you did to cause them and try not to do it again. If you know you are going to eat a big meal, you might take digestive enzymes. This might help the situation.

Corticosteroids

The long-term use of corticosteroids is another bone calcium robber. Corticosteroids are prescription drugs used when inflammation becomes a problem, such as in arthritis or asthma. The overall effect of corticosteroids is to inhibit gastro-intestinal intake of calcium and slightly decrease calcium being put back in the bones. Rarely is there a change in the blood levels of calcium because the parathyroid glands pull calcium from the bones to help keep the blood in homeostasis. There is also increased urinary secretion of calcium at this time. The long-term use of corticosteroids can have a disastrous effect on the bones.

Prednisone is one of the corticosteroids known to inhibit the intestinal absorption of calcium. Gentamicin and tobramycin can also cause an excess of magnesium in the urine. Excess calcium in the urine occurs after long-term use of corticosteroids such as aldosterone. Clearly, corticosteroids upset the minerals and the whole body chemistry.

To find out the effect of the use of corticosteroids by asthmatics, 128 patients, all over forty years of age who had taken steroids for at least a year, were compared to 54 asthmatics of similar age who had not required long-term administration of steroids. The researchers found a total of fifty-eight fractures of ribs or vertebrae in 14 of the patients who had received long-term steroid treatment (11 percent) and no evidence of fractures in the patients who had not received long-term treatment. The researchers concluded that long-term steroid therapy in asthmatic patients is associated with a decrease in the trabecular (innermost part) bone density. There was also an increased prevalence of rib and vertebral fractures.

Calcium Blockers or Beta Blockers

Calcium blockers or beta blockers are a new class of drugs designed to keep calcium out of the cells. Calcium is normally found in the fluid of the blood; very little is found in the cells. Extracellular calcium levels are typically 1,000 to 10,000 times greater than the levels of intracellular calcium. Our cells don't like to have too much calcium in them; it keeps them from functioning well.

However, when the body chemistry becomes upset due to an increase or decrease in phosphorus, the functioning calcium level in the blood drops. This causes generalized bone mineralization, which means minerals are pulled out of the bone. Frequently, some of the calcium pulled out becomes toxic and gets into cells and tissues, causing problems. It also appears that excess calcium in arteries, joints, and tissues may be indirectly related to the generalized demineralization of bones. The excess accumulation of calcium in the cells of the arteries is a major contributor to cardiovascular disease.

Besides helping to digest food, enzymes do many other jobs in our bodies. One of these jobs is removing calcium from cells, but this can only happen when the body can maintain homeostasis. When the body chemistry is upset, the enzymes do not function well enough to rid the cells of excess calcium. Drugs such as beta blockers are called in to do the job. But rather than taking a drug to block calcium in the cells, it seems more logical to stop upsetting the body chemistry so that the calcium won't get into the cells in the first place.

Drugs should be for crisis medicine, not for long-term use. The long-term use of most drugs can cause side effects such as liver disorders, hypoglycemia, and stomach problems, as well as osteoporosis. Teen-agers who are on long-term use of antibiotics for skin problems should be made aware of these possible dangers in later life. Lifestyle changes can often prove to be better options. Junk food should be eliminated from their diets; it is often the cause of pimples. The arthritic should find out what foods are causing the pain (see fasting on page 26) and what role stress plays in the disease process. Stop upsetting the body chemistry and the drugs will no longer be necessary.

The medical community keeps coming up with arthritic drugs that are supposed to be miraculous, and then they are taken off the market because of side effects. The health community keeps coming up with supplements that are supposed to be the answer to our problems: yeast, garlic, pau d'arco tea, Vitamin E, fish oils, germanium, co-enzyme Q, and boron. But the answer is much simpler: just stop doing what you did to upset your body chemistry and the body will heal itself.

The July 12, 1990, issue of the *New England Journal of Medicine* reports on the effects of the drug etidronate. In a two-year study, it was reported that this drug reduced the vertebral fractures in post-menopausal women by 50 percent, while increasing the spinal bone density by an average of 4 to 5 percent. At the time of the writing of *Healthy Bones*, etidronate has not yet been approved for osteoporosis by the United States Government. It is still in the experimental stages, and the long-term side effects are still unknown; however, it is a drug worth keeping an eye on. Personally, I do not believe there are any magic pills or potions. I stand by my conviction that it is far better to get your body into the balanced state of homeostasis and let it heal.

Fluoridation

The fluoridation of our water supply, our toothpaste, and sometimes even our teeth has long been a controversial subject. It has been called everything from an essential service of public health to a communist plot. I am convinced after considering all the available research that the effect of fluorides on the body chemistry is far worse than any beneficial effects they might have.

Fluorides have one of the most avid affinities for other elements of any substance known to man. They grasp calcium and remove it from the system, depriving the body of calcium and replacing it with sodium. Fluorine, which comes from fluoridated water supplies, has been found to carry magnesium out of the body.

Dr. Hugo Theorell, winner of the 1958 Nobel Prize for his work with enzymes, found that fluorides inhibit and destroy vital enzymes, the chemical activators essential for digestion and most other vital life functions. For this reason, he recommended that Sweden outlaw fluoridation, and that it did.

Fluoretic bone is denser and more brittle than normal bone, and its structure is irregular. There may be other long-term side effects of fluoride supplements that have not yet come to light. What might happen to cells exposed to high concentrations of fluoride? We don't know. But it seems clear that extra fluoride in any form should be avoided. Keep your body chemistry in balance, and the problem of osteoporosis will be minimal.

Intravenous Feeding

Many times after an operation, a patient cannot eat because his or her gastro-intestinal tract is not functioning optimally.

The doctor administers calories through intravenous feeding (IV) of sugar (dextrose), and sometimes vitamins, minerals, fats, and amino acids. These are diluted with water and dripped into the arm of the patient until the gastro-intestinal tract is functioning again. At that point the IV is no longer needed and the patient can eat by mouth again.

This form of feeding is called *total parenteral nutrition* (TPN). It is given to patients recovering from operations, and also to those with bowel diseases and gastro-intestinal problems. Mothers who have just given birth and newborn babies also receive TPN in many hospitals.

Recently, parenteral nutrition has been the subject of much research. The findings show that in as little as three months, people on TPN can have such intense lower back pain that they can become wheelchair bound. This insidious onset of bone pain is very severe and causes considerable disability. As a result, patients are more apt to become dependent on narcotics. In addition to the pain, a patchy osteomalacia may start to appear. Osteomalacia is a sponginess of the bones that is usually a forerunner to osteoporosis. But when the TPN was discontinued and normal feeding resumed, the pain was gone within two months.

Patients are given sugar intravenously for the calories it contains, so that they will not lose weight. If you need to have an IV and are not underweight, I suggest that you consult with your doctor about the possibility of leaving the sugar out and receiving just the vitamins, minerals, fats, and amino acids. It will be more nutritious and less disruptive to your body chemistry.

Heavy Metals

Research has demonstrated that chronic exposure to heavy metals such as lead, cadmium, mercury, and aluminum in our water, food, and air contributes to excess intracellular accumulation of calcium. As I said earlier, excess calcium does not belong in cells. This amounts to an upset body chemistry.

Aluminum is difficult to avoid because it is present in antacids, salt, baking powder, non-dairy creamers, cake and pancake mixes, frozen dough, processed cheese, toothpaste, deodorant, anti-diarrhea products, and buffered aspirin. Aluminum in pots and pans can also be leached out when acidic foods, such as tomatoes and rhubarb, are cooked in them.

Aluminum-containing drugs bind onto most of the phosphorus available in the intestines and carry it away in the stool. Phosphorus is also lost in the urine. The body's phosphorus stores become depleted whenever aluminum-containing drugs are taken regularly for a long time.

Most of the phosphorus is held in our bones where, in combination with calcium, it provides them with strength and rigidity. Thus, when phosphorus is lost from the body, the bones become weakened and easily fractured. When the phosphorus becomes depleted, the calcium is also unable to function, since all minerals work in relation to one another.

You don't hear much about cadmium, but it is probably one of the most dangerous of the heavy metals. Cadmium is especially dangerous because our bodies accept it in place of zinc. In other words, if enough zinc is not available during some chemical chain of events occurring in our bodies, cadmium steps in and fills the spot. Unfortunately, the chemical process comes to a halt.

Besides being present in cigarette smoke (see page 51), cadmium is leached out of galvanized pipes by acidic water, hot water, and especially soft water. If you are still drinking tap water, don't drink the first water out of the tap in the morning; let it run a short time first. When possible, use cold water for your cooking.

Another major source of cadmium is white flour. Cadmium is distributed throughout the grain of wheat. Zinc, on the other hand, is concentrated in the germ and the bran. Processing the flour removes the zinc and concentrates the cadmium. Processed flour has six times more cadmium than zinc. Go back to natural foods. This is just one good example of what processing does to food.

Overeating

Even if you don't abuse your body with the foods and non-foods that have just been discussed, you can still exhaust the metabolic pathways and secrete calcium by overeating at any one time. Your digestive system has only so many enzymes, and your buffer systems have a certain capacity. When you exhaust these by eating too much at one meal, you're in for trouble. A loss of calcium can be the end result.

So, don't eat too much of one food at one time, don't eat too much food at one meal, don't eat too much protein, don't eat over-processed foods, and don't overcook your food. That is enough of "don'ts." In the next chapter, I will present some "do's" that can help you adopt a healthy lifestyle.

4 | Balancing Act

The bad news is that an upset body chemistry can result in osteoporosis as well as other diseases and deterioration. Now for the good news: all of these diseases are preventable and many are reversible. Just stop upsetting mineral relationships and the body will heal itself.

All of us can bring our bodies back to balance, to homeostasis. How long it takes to obtain and maintain homeostasis is individual to each of us. It depends upon our genetic blueprints, how much stress we live with on a daily basis, how much junk food we have eaten in the past and how much we are eating right now, how old we are, and other factors. Some people remain out of homeostasis for a long period of time each time they upset their body chemistries. Others balance back quickly.

I believe all disease is preventable. If you have a disease such as arthritis, you can stop the disease process and remove such symptoms as joint pain and stiffness. If the disease process has led to tissue damage, as you might see in arthritic fingers, it is difficult to reverse, although I have seen miracles.

Dr. Melvin Page, a dentist, helped his clients who had periodontal disease obtain homeostasis through stress reduction and diet change. After the body had been in homeostasis for a period of time, the periodontal disease went away. The gums no longer receded, the pockets no longer formed, and Page actually saw bone growth in the mouth. If bone can grow in the mouth, it seems obvious that it can grow in other parts of the body as well.

Diet

So, what should you eat to prevent or stop osteoporosis? Actually, what you don't put in your mouth is more important than what you do. Don't eat all of those foods and non-foods discussed in Chapter 3. They will lead to osteoporosis.

To obtain optimal nutrition, it is best to eat small amounts of a variety of evolutionary foods. These are foods that our ancestors ate; foods that we have the evolutionary enzymes to digest; foods that don't upset the body chemistry. Eat a variety of vegetables, beans, grains, and small amounts of protein. The food plans offered in Chapter 5 have all the vitamins, minerals, amino acids (protein), fatty acids, and carbohydrates needed for good health.

The key is to keep yourself in homeostasis. If you feel well and a urine test (order form in back of book) shows that you are in balance, then continue eating and doing what you are doing. If you don't feel well and you do not maintain homeostasis, look to your lifestyle to see what could be upsetting that balance.

Each of us is different. We all have different genetic blueprints, we each deal with stress differently, some of us eat more sugar than others, some exercise more, and we are all different ages. When we do abuse our bodies, some of us balance back to homeostasis readily, while others do not. Because of these differences, I have offered three different food plans in Chapter 5.

These food plans can help you obtain and maintain homeostasis. Some of you will only have to eat in accordance with Food Plan I. Others will need to follow a stricter diet and use Food Plan II or III. This is a time to listen to your body, to get in touch with what it is telling you. Your body talks to you all the time, so you must listen. Symptoms are warnings that all is not well inside, and it is up to you to figure out their causes. These food plans should help. Foods from Food Plan III are those that upset the body chemistry of healthy people the least.

Calcium

If you are wondering where you will get your calcium, do not fret. When the body is in homeostasis, it absorbs all of the nutrients from the food that is ingested. When it is not in balance, it has a difficult time absorbing the nutrients; many are not absorbed and/or are excreted in the urine.

According to the World Health Organization (WHO), we need only 500 milligrams of calcium per day. I believe this to be correct, but only if the body is in homeostasis. If the body is not in homeostasis, then even the 1,000 milligrams or more that the United States Food and Drug Administration (FDA) says we should have will not be absorbed. Osteoporosis is becoming an enormous problem, but taking more calcium is not the answer.

There is considerable evidence showing that we really don't need the 1,000 or more milligrams of calcium a day that the Nutritional Academy of Sciences—National Research Council suggests. This group, which is responsible for determining dietary standards, readily admits that many individuals and populations consume much lower intakes of calcium than those recommended, yet do so apparently without ill effects.

In most developing countries, where a relatively low intake of milk products is the norm, the total daily intake of calcium is habitually low. Among South African Bantu, investigations have revealed that probably less than 5 percent ingest 500 milligrams or more of calcium a day, the general range of intake being 175–475 milligrams per day.

Researchers studied the Bantu to see if there were any adverse effects with respect to growth; pregnancy and lactation; bone composition, density, and dimension; prevalence of dental caries, rickets, osteomalacia, and osteoporosis; and nonskeletal processes in which calcium is involved. The conclusions of the researchers seemed to be that there was no evidence that a habitually low intake of calcium is detrimental to man, or that an increase in calcium intake would result in clinically detectable benefits.

I have read some interesting information on calcium intake and absorption during pregnancy and lactation. First, increased absorption of calcium has been documented in both pregnant and lactating animals. This means that the calcium that pregnant and lactating women take is absorbed and utilized better. Secondly, research showed that repeated pregnancies and lactations produced no evidence of bone loss, even in women consuming only 320 milligrams of calcium per day.

There is also no evidence that calcium supplements, taken either in pregnancy or during lactation, have benefits for the women as compared with a control group not receiving supplements. The best thing a mother can do for a fetus or newborn baby (if breast-feeding) is to eat well and deal with stress well. Keeping the body in homeostasis is far more important than taking a lot of supplements. Taking supplements when the body is out of homeostasis is not useful either.

I recently traveled in Indonesia, a country where people use very little milk or milk products in their diets. In fact, on some of the islands, there are no fresh dairy products available at all—no milk, butter, or cheese, except at hotels that cater to tourists, and then the butter comes from Australia. Living conditions in Indonesia are very primitive. White rice is the mainstay of the diet. A few beans, tofu, tempura, vegetables, and small amounts of beef, chicken, or fish are added to the rice to vary the taste.

The average person in Indonesia lives to age fifty-five, but this figure is deceiving. The reason that the average age of death is so low is because 12.5 percent of babies die at birth. There are many older people in Indonesia. I did not see any older or younger men or women with any signs of osteoporosis—none. So here is a population that has older men and women, consumes no milk products, takes no estrogen or calcium supplements, and are small people with small bones. Yet, they do not have osteoporosis. Admittedly, my research is limited, but after spending time in many different villages and cities, talking to health officials and people who worked in hospitals, and learning birth and death statistics, I feel that these facts are quite accurate.

The average household in Indonesia contains six to ten children. Pregnant and lactating women do not take extra calcium, yet there is still no osteoporosis. The difference is that these people do not eat sugar, eat very little protein at one meal, drink very small amounts of alcohol, and consume only small amounts of caffeine. They do drink tea, but not coffee. They also use very few antibiotics, corticosteroids, or antacids. The women still carry baskets on their heads to and from markets, so exercise still plays an important role in their lifestyle.

In the local *apotecs* (pharmacies), I did see a lot of different antihistamines used by people with allergies. Sadly, this indicated that they are at the first stage of the degenerative disease process, allergies. They will go on to more debilitating diseases as "civilization" continues to invade their country. My heart skipped a beat when I saw women carrying food from the market, the baskets on their heads loaded with soft drinks. Coca-Cola increased its sales in Indonesia by 21 percent in the second quarter of 1988. Colonel Sanders was the first of the fast-food chains to arrive.

Some people have argued that because we live in Western society with its excess protein, alcohol, drugs, and caffeine, we need to take extra calcium. I do not believe that at all. I believe that as long as we upset our body chemistries and continually stress ourselves, it won't matter how much calcium we take. It just won't help. This may sound radical, but all evidence points to this position.

Two researchers, Heaney and Recker, found interesting information after studying 171 early post-menopausal women whose average age was fifty-three. What they found was that absorption of calcium in 55 percent of the women was inadequate if they were to maintain mineral balance on a recommended intake of calcium of 800 milligrams a day. These researchers go on to say that they predicted positive calcium balance could not be maintained in 75 percent of the women, even at an intake of 1.5 grams (1,500 milligrams) of calcium a day. The researchers concluded that the basis for low absorption performance in this group was defective absorption.

Of course, these researchers did not study how much sugar or other refined foods these women were eating. They might call it defective absorption, but I would say if the women had been eating only fruits, vegetables, grains, and protein, the "defective absorption" would not have been so defective. The major problem with research today is the difficulty in controlling the total diet when studying one food item. In order to control the total diet, a research group needs to be put in a hospital or other institution.

If you have a group of people taking 1,500 milligrams of calcium a day through food, they might take some of it with a fruit yogurt. Unfortunately, most fruit yogurts contain seven teaspoons of sugar per cup. Taking a fruit yogurt and then studying the absorption of calcium would be impossible due to the sugar.

I remember one study, which excited me because of its strict controls; I thought it would be a valid study. The article started by saying, "All studies were carried out on a metabolic ward, using a complete balanced regimen, and most employed a liquid formula diet of fixed composition." Unfortunately, it went on to say, " . . . supplemented with graham crackers or shortbread cookies." This study, then, had little validity.

As long as you eat a natural diet that includes vegetables, beans, grains, and small amounts of protein, you will get all the calcium you need. Add caffeine, alcohol, antacids, drugs, sugar, or refined food, however, and it won't matter how natural the rest of the diet is. The calcium from the natural diet will be less available to the cells because the abusive substances will upset the body chemistry. Table 4.1 presents specific information on calcium found in common foods.

There is no discrepancy between medical practitioners, scientists, researchers, and me that osteoporosis is caused by a deficiency in calcium. It is on how this deficiency develops that we disagree. We also seem to agree that when there is a deficiency of estrogen, osteoporosis can develop. Since estrogen is secreted by one of the endocrine glands, we want to make sure that our endocrine glands are functioning optimally.

To make sure your endocrine glands are working optimally, get your body in homeostasis and keep it there. The calcium will absorb more readily and osteoporosis will not be a problem. In women, this will allow the ovaries to secrete as much estrogen as they are capable of. I will not discuss the pros and cons of taking synthetic estrogen. This is a subject you might discuss with your doctor.

Consuming more calcium will not solve any problems. As we saw in Chapter 3, excess calcium can become nonfunctioning or toxic and play havoc in the bloodstream. Nevertheless, many products today are calcium-fortified. Extra cal-

Table 4.1   Calcium and Common Foods

Food	Amount	Calcium Content (milligrams)
VEGETABLES		
Bok choy	1 cup (cooked)	250
Broccoli	1 cup	190
Brussels sprouts	1 cup	50
Cabbage	1 cup	34
Cabbage	1 cup (cooked)	64
Carrots	1 cup	45
Celery pieces	1 cup (cooked)	39
Collard greens	1 cup (cooked)	289
Kale	1 cup	210
Mustard greens	1 cup (cooked)	193
Spinach	1 cup	200
Squash	1 cup (cooked)	55
Sweet potatoes	1 medium	52
Turnip greens	1 cup (cooked)	252
FISH		
Bluefish	3 ounces	244
Crabmeat	1 cup	246
Haddock	3 ounces	210
Mackerel	4 ounces (canned)	300
Oysters	4 ounces (canned)	100
Oysters	4 ounces (raw)	110
Salmon, pink	4 ounces (canned)	220
Salmon, red	4 ounces (canned)	290
Sardines, oil-packed	4 ounces (canned)	500
Scallops	4 ounces	130
Shrimp	4 ounces	130
Tuna, oil-packed	3 ounces	199
BEANS		
Kidney	1 cup	74
Lima	1 cup	63
Navy	1 cup	100
Soy	1 cup (cooked)	138
Tofu	1/4 ounce	145
NUTS		
Almonds	1/2 cup	160

Food	Amount	Calcium Content (milligrams)
Pecans	½ cup	42
Walnuts	½ cup	50
MISCELLANEOUS		
Blackberries	½ cup	46
Oranges	1 medium	54
Peanuts	½ cup	107
Whole wheat bread	1 slice	22

Reprinted with permission of Macmillan Publishing Company from *Principles of Nutrition* by Wilson, Eva D., Fisher, Katherine H., and Garcia, Pilar A. Copyright © 1979.

cium is being added to orange juice, bread, soft drinks, milk, and yogurt. It will be difficult to tell how much calcium you are getting. It seems to me that Mother Nature did a pretty good job of balancing the nutrients in natural foods. Why tinker with the real thing?

Boron

In an article from the November 1989 issue of *Longevity*, some interesting facts on the trace mineral boron were presented.

Researchers at the United States Department of Agriculture's Human Nutrition Center in Grand Forks, North Dakota, found that boron, a trace mineral found in the soil, may be essential to calcium metabolism. In 1986, nutritional biochemist Forrest H. Neilsen, Ph.D., and colleagues at the center began human studies. Twelve post-menopausal women were put on a very low boron diet (0.25 milligrams a day) for seventeen weeks. Then the researchers kept these people on the same diet, but added a daily 3-milligram boron supplement, for another seven weeks. Within eight days of starting the boron supplement, the women excreted 40 percent less calcium in their urine. This calcium loss was less than when they ate normally.

Neilsen came to an interesting conclusion about boron deficiency. He realized that even though Americans were eating generous amounts of calcium-rich dairy products and taking calcium supplements, they were still getting osteoporosis. He didn't realize that all minerals work in relationship to each other and if the boron was deficient, there were probably many other minerals that were deficient, also. He did realize, however, that if the boron was low, then the calcium consumed might not be assimilated and metabolized and would become deficient.

During a four-month follow-up study of fifteen people, his conclusions were confirmed. He varied the amount of boron given to this control group and found that this alone affected the body's ability to retain calcium.

What Neilsen didn't realize was that even though a person might be getting enough boron in his diet, if he continued to eat sugar or upset his body chemistry in other ways, the boron, calcium, and other minerals would be less available to the body.

So where do you get boron? The best sources of boron are in legumes (peas and beans), leafy green vegetables, nuts, and non-citrus fruits (especially apples, grapes, and pears). Food Plans II and III (found in Chapter 5) are good to follow if you are interested in getting boron into your diet.

Use It or Lose It

Exercise is the only way, short of potent medication, to significantly increase bone mass after you have stopped growing. As with muscles, stress (not distress) strengthens bones. One study showed that those who exercised for one hour, three times a week, for one year actually gained bone mass, whereas a comparison group of sedentary women lost bone mass.

Peter Jacobbson and associates at the University of North Carolina, Chapel Hill, tested 80 women ranging in age from 35 to 65 who played tennis three times weekly against 400 sedentary women in the same age brackets. Tennis players in the 35–55 age group had no more bone than the control group, just as the scientists had suspected, because bone loss is uncommon before menopause. But tennis players in the 55–65 age bracket had far more bone than the sedentary women.

In another study, a group of 14 post-menopausal women exercised three times a week for fifty minutes for five months. This group was compared with 26 inactive women on three occasions: one year prior to the study, at the beginning of the study, and at the end. During the year preceding the exercise program, the mean bone density decreased significantly in both groups. During the exercise period, the bone density of the exercise group increased 3.8 percent, while that of the control group continued to decline. This study demonstrated that an appropriate physical activity regime may be effective as a treatment for post-menopausal bone loss.

There is a basic principle known as Wolf's Law that states that bones respond to stress. If you were to hop on your right leg for the next couple of weeks, the bone in the right leg would get stronger and appear more dense on x-rays. At the same time, the left leg, which would not have had any weight on it, would weaken. If a bone is stressed (not distressed), it will become stronger.

Studies have shown that the bones in the dominant arm of a professional tennis player are denser than those in the other arm. The repetitive, vigorous use and pull of muscles have indeed strengthened these bones.

There is a common misunderstanding connecting running with bone problems. Many people believe that osteoarthritis and osteoporosis can be caused by running. Our bodies were made to be used, not abused, but running is not an abuse; it is a use.

Nancy Lane and her colleagues reported on a study in which the bone status of forty-one long-distance runners (male and female) between fifty and seventy-two years of age was assessed. The results were compared to an equal number of matched controls and showed no evidence of the development of osteoarthritis in response to repetitive long-term running.

These results are supported by a study conducted by R. S. Panush and colleagues who could not find any evidence of long-term running as the cause of degenerative joint disease of the lower extremities in men. No significant differences were found between seventeen runners (mean age fifty-six years, running an average of twenty-eight miles per week for twelve years) and eighteen non-runners for reported musculoskeletal complaints; swelling or pain in the hips, knees, ankles, or feet; or for radiological evidence of degeneration or cartilage thickness. Upset body chemistry causes osteoarthritis and osteoporosis, not running.

The best kind of exercise for healthy bones is weight-bearing exercise. Walking, hiking, climbing, jogging, running, bicycling, rope jumping, tennis, basketball, dancing, and aerobics are all excellent ways to prevent or slow bone loss. According to the *Mayo Clinic Proceedings*, it has been discovered that the density and amount of calcium in an older woman's spinal bones correlates very closely to the strength of her back muscles. It is a wise idea to do exercises that tone up these muscles.

These research papers and others seem to indicate that each of us should be exercising a minimum of fifty minutes, three times a week. If you don't exercise now, start slowly and explore a variety of activities. Find ones that you like. If you don't like doing the exercise, chances are you will quit.

I live in Santa Monica, California, and aside from playing tennis, one of my favorite sports is climbing the Santa Monica steps. There are 190 of them, and I do the steps ten times. I started with two sets about two years ago and slowly advanced to ten sets, twice a week. I feel great when I'm finished!

All this physical activity is also helpful for many other body functions. Any exercise that includes aerobics helps with cardiovascular function. Deep breathing helps oxygen uptake and lung function. All forms of exercise help with stress reduction and can be fun, too.

However, it's important to realize that exercise is not a miracle cure. For one thing, too much of it can be as bad as none at all. According to Henry A. Soloman, M. D., cardiologist at Cornell University Medical College, "Young women who exercise to extremes and reduce their body fat level to 10–15 percent seem to trigger hormonal changes that alter their regular menstrual cycles and cause calcium loss. This applies to any actively menstruating woman, though most of the cases that have been seen are women in their twenties and thirties."

Young women who stop menstruating because of intense exercise, emotional stress, or other unnatural reasons face a greater risk of having brittle bones when they get older. Studies show that anorexics who exercise and fast retain more bone mass than those who only fast, but neither group gets adequate dietary calcium.

Evidence supports the following conclusions on the relationship between bones and exercise:

- Exercise beginning at an early age causes maximum mineral content in the bones at maturity. This is important because when bones reach maturity, the normal loss of bone mass begins. Therefore, the greater the mineral content found in the bones, the greater the amount retained at a later age.
- The onset of bone mineral loss is delayed by physical activity during adulthood.
- The rate of bone mineral loss, once commenced, can be reduced by physical activity.

Even if you don't over-exercise or under-exercise, exercise is not the only answer. You could be doing all the exercising necessary, but still get osteoporosis if your body chemistry is upset. Remember to keep your body in homeostasis. That is the most important thing of all.

Body Language

When your body chemistry is upset, your body will usually give you signals. These signals are telling you that your body is not in homeostasis and you could be pulling calcium from the bones. The following are some examples of signals or symptoms telling you that all is not well in your body after you have eaten. These reactions can be immediate or delayed.

Immediate reactions:

- feeling much better*
- feeling lousy*
- sleepiness
- fatigue
- gas
- bloating
- headache
- dizziness
- irritability
- diarrhea

*You shouldn't feel noticeably better or worse after eating. You should feel the same.

Delayed reactions:

- constipation
- diarrhea
- joint pains
- muscle cramps
- headache
- arthritis
- rashes or other skin disorders
- irritability

When you notice these signals, try to figure out what is wrong, what you are doing to upset your body chemistry, and then stop. I have given you suggestions as to what could be causing these upsets. You have a responsibility to be your own detective. The urine test for homeostasis and calcium secretion is very helpful. You can order this test with the form found in the back of this book.

Survival Techniques

We live in the twentieth century with fast foods, freeways, smog, jobs that are too far away, broken families, and hundreds of subcultures that pull us in many different directions. These are the facts. The most important thing is to remember that it is not life's situations that cause the problems, but how we deal with them that makes or breaks our arteries, our bones, our bodies. None of us is without problems. It can be just as stressful for one person to decide which job to take as it is for another to decide whether or not to institutionalize a parent. Distress is the biggest cause of osteoporosis today. So first and foremost, you must learn to deal with the stress in your life. Coping is the key.

Statistically, every week, each working person eats approximately eleven meals in restaurants. Fast-food restaurants are not only getting faster, larger, and greater in number in the United States, but around the world as well. However, there is a light at the end of the tunnel. Fast-food restaurants exist to make money, and many are discovering if they want to continue making money, they had better give the public what it wants. As more and more people are becoming aware of food quality, more demands are being made on restaurants.

Most fast food places today still have the fried hamburgers, milkshakes, soft drinks, and french fries, but are also offering a variety of salads, salad bars, baked potatoes, and chili with beans. In addition, salad bars and salad counters with a variety of "to go" salads can be found in many of our national grocery stores.

With a little planning, you can eat almost anywhere and not be deprived. When I eat in restaurants, I bring my own herbal tea bags and just ask for hot water. Sometimes I take a small jar (baby food or vitamin jar) of salad dressing with me and say, "Hold the salad dressing," when ordering a salad.

I continually ask questions at restaurants of the waiters and waitresses. Are the foods prepared with margarine or butter? (Always prefer what nature has made to what man has made.) Is that non-dairy creamer or half-and-half? Do you fry your fish or broil it? Are the vegetables canned, frozen, or fresh? Do you use sulfites on your salads? Are the potatoes from packages or are they the real thing? Do you boil your vegetables or steam them? Do you have a non-smoking section? Even if you know the restaurant does not have a non-smoking section, make your point by asking anyway.

If the restaurant does not have good soundproof ceilings and walls, if it has a TV that is blaring, or plays loud rock music, I might try another restaurant. At a hotel, I ask for a non-smoking room. I test the beds, listen to the noises from the surrounding rooms, and ask for another room if all is not satisfactory.

Another thing I do is ask my doctor questions. Years ago, I played the game—if he didn't discover something from a blood test or didn't ask me the right questions, I wasn't going to volunteer any information. Now I have a list of questions of my own. When he says my blood test is fine, I tell him I want to know more. I learned how to read one myself. I always ask for a copy of my tests and keep them on file at home.

If I do get sick and a drug is prescribed, I do my homework. I have a book dealing with the side effects of prescription drugs, and I consult it. I also ask my pharmacist for the information sheet that comes with every drug. This warns of the drug's possible side effects and includes a list of drugs that should not be taken together.

If I agree to go on antibiotics, I make sure I go to a health food store and purchase a bottle of acidophilus to take with it. Antibiotics kill off the good and the bad bacteria. Acidophilus helps bring back the bacteria our bodies need, making us less susceptible to yeast infections and other problems.

It's also a good idea to read all the latest information in the health field. New research and suggestions are given out all the time. One of my favorite magazines in *Longevity*, but there are many others besides. Go to a health food store and you will see that the list is endless.

All of these survival techniques can help you take charge of your life and avoid disease.

5 | A Happy Ending

I believe that each one of us has the ability to create health or disease, to have osteoporosis or not to have it. It is up to us. We are responsible for our own health. When we learn to deal creatively with the stress in our lives, eat natural foods that enhance homeostasis, remove those foods that upset body chemistry, and make exercise a part of our weekly routine, our bodies will function optimally and disease will be at a minimum. We will go into our older years without degenerative diseases.

You have been given ideas on exercise, stress reduction, and what not to eat. What follows in this chapter are food plans, healthy eating suggestions, and recipes.

Food Plan I is for healthy people who want an optimal diet. Food Plan II is for those who have symptoms and are not in homeostasis continually while following Food Plan I. Food Plan III is for those suffering from osteoporosis or any other degenerative disease.

Remember, these food plans are not diets, but are ways of eating for the rest of your life. Listen to your body for symptoms, and periodically test your body for homeostasis to find out which food plan is best for you.

You, alone, are responsible for the foods that go into your mouth, for the words that come out of your mouth, and for what you think and feel. Although one out of every two people will die of heart disease, and one out of every three people will get cancer, I don't believe we need to spend any part of our lives with osteoporosis, diabetes, arthritis, or any other degenerative disease.

Do you know what the average 100-year-old person dies of? Nothing. He wills himself to live and he wills himself to die. I believe all of us can do the same thing.

Food Plans

The following food plans are effective particularly when used in conjunction with the Body Chemistry Kit (order form found in back of book).

CAUTION: Following Food Plans, I, II, or III may initiate withdrawal symptoms and a phenomenon called physiological and psychological detox. You may experience different symptoms, many similar to withdrawal from any addiction. Fever, depression, headaches, chills, and fatigue are the most common symptoms.

Food Plan I

1. Avoid all foods in Categories IV and V (see food lists starting on page 96). Eat any other food.
2. If after being on this plan for seven days, you are not feeling better, your body chemistry requires a more com-

prehensive food plan. Therefore, proceed with Food Plan II.

Food Plan II

1. Avoid all foods in Categories III, IV, and V, and eat foods in Category II only in small amounts and only between meals. For meals, eat Category I foods.
2. If after being on Plan II for seven days, you are still not experiencing better health, you need to proceed to Food Plan III.

Food Plan III

It is clear that your unbalanced body chemistry involves more than just the foods common to body chemistry upset.

Food Plan III is designed to provide complete nutrients to your body in their most bio-available form. Adherence to this plan automatically handles some complex food-related biochemical problems that Food Plans I and II did not handle. The procedures and foods of Food Plan III are the least stressful to your body chemistry.

1. For the next fourteen days eat only foods from Category I. Eat one small portion from each food group four or five times a day. Remember to follow the Health-Promoting Eating Habits found on page 101.
2. If after fourteen days you are still not experiencing relief of symptoms, you'll need to see a qualified practitioner who can give you blood tests and a test for food sensitivities, and can help you to find foods that do not upset your body chemistry.

Food Categories

Category I

When prepared and eaten in a proper manner, the foods of Category I are tolerated best by the already unbalanced body chemistry of people with health breakdowns.

Group 1

GREEN LEAFY VEGETABLES

Artichoke
Brussels sprouts
Cabbage
Kale
Lettuce (all)
Spinach

Group 2

GREEN VEGETABLES

Alfalfa
Asparagus
Avocado
Broccoli
Celery
Chinese pea
Okra

Group 3

YELLOW/WHITE VEGETABLES

Cauliflower
Corn
Cucumber
Squash (all)

Group 4

ROOT VEGETABLES

Jicama
Onion
Parsnip
Potato
Radish
Rutabaga
Turnip

Group 5

ORANGE/PURPLE/ RED VEGETABLES

Beet
Carrot
Eggplant
Pumpkin
Sweet potato
Tomato

HERBS/ CONDIMENTS

Arrowroot
Basil
Bay leaf
Black pepper
Butter
Caraway
Chili pepper
Chive
Cilantro
Dill
Garlic
Ginger
Horseradish
Lemon
Lime
Mustard
Nutmeg
Olive oil
Oregano
Parsley
Rose hip
Rosemary
Safflower oil
Sage
Sesame oil
Sunflower oil
Tarragon
Thyme

Group 6   *Group 7*

FISH	MEAT/POULTRY	BEANS/GRAINS
Anchovy		Azuki bean
Bass	Bacon	Barley
Catfish	Beef	Bean sprout
Clam	Chicken	Black bean
Cod	Chicken egg	Black-eyed pea
Crab	Duck	Buckwheat
Founder	Frog's leg	Garbanzo bean
Haddock	Lamb	Green pea
Halibut	Liver, beef	Kidney bean
Mackerel	Liver, chicken	Lentil
Oyster	Pheasant	Lima bean
Perch	Pork	Millet
Red snapper	Turkey	Navy bean
Salmon	Venison	Oat
Sardine		Pinto bean
Scallop		Red bean
Shark		Rice, brown
Shrimp		Rice, white
Sole		Rice, wild
Swordfish		Rye
Trout		Soybean
Tuna		Split pea
Any other fish		String bean
		White bean

If you are a vegetarian, use our Food Plans, but eliminate Group 6 and combine your beans and grains in Group 7 to give complete protein.

Category II

Certain areas of some people's body chemistry have become sensitive to these otherwise wholesome foods.

FRUITS	NUTS/SEEDS	HERBS/ CONDIMENTS
Apple	Almond	Allspice
Apricot	Brazil nut	Anise seed
Avocado	Chestnut	Chicory
Banana	Flax seed	Clove
Cantaloupe	Hazelnut	Cream of tartar
Coconut	Hickory nut	Paprika
Cranberry	Macadamia nut	Spearmint
Date	Pecan	
Fig	Pistachio	
Grape	Poppy seed	
Guava	Safflower seed	
Melon (all)	Sunflower seed	
Nectarine	Walnut	
Papaya		
Peach		
Pear		
Pineapple		
Plum (prune)		
Raspberry		
Strawberry		
Watermelon		

Category III

Overcooking, overeating, and eating with sugar have turned these normally well-tolerated foods into potentially abusive foods. These foods can now unbalance the chemistry of those who have already impaired their ability to rebalance their body chemistry.

YEAST
Baker's yeast
Brewer's yeast
Mushrooms

GRAINS
Wheat bran
Wheat germ
White flour
Whole wheat

FRUITS
Grapefruit
Mango
Orange
Tangerine

HERBS
Curry
Peppermint
Salt
Vanilla

DAIRY
Blue cheese
Buttermilk
Cheese (all)
Cottage cheese
Cow's milk
Cream cheese
Whey
Yogurt

NUTS/SEEDS
Cashew
Peanut

MISCELLANEOUS
Carob
Cinnamon
Coffee
Coffee, decaf.
Cola bean
Corn gluten
Cornstarch
Fructose
Honey
Hops
Molasses
Tea

Category IV

These foods are always abusive to human body chemistry. Only those who remain adaptive can rebalance their body chemistry after frequent exposure to Category IV foods. The more Category IV foods consumed, the more rapid the deterioration in the body chemistry.

Alcohol
Beet sugar
Cane sugar

Cocoa
Corn sugar
Corn syrup

Malt
Maple sugar
Saccharin

Category V

These chemicals have known unbalancing effects on the body chemistry, and it serves your health to use them seldom and with caution.

Aspirin	Food coloring	Tobacco
Baking powder	Formaldehyde	Tylenol
BHT	MSG	Sodium benzoate
Caffeine	Petroleum by-products	

Simple Suggestions for Breakfasts and Snacks

People who are on Food Plan III, and eat only Category I foods, sometimes have difficulty with ideas for breakfast. Here are a few suggestions, many of which can also be used for snacks.

1. Bake potatoes the night before and refrigerate. In the morning slice potatoes and sauté in butter at a low temperature.
2. Baked potato with butter, guacamole, or puréed beans.
3. Corn tortilla with butter, tomatoes, an egg, and/or guacamole.
4. Oatmeal with butter.
5. Cream of Rice with butter.
6. Rice cakes with sliced avocado, tomato, onion, green pepper, or cucumber.
7. One-egg omelet with sliced tomato, cut-up potato, green pepper, onion, or other vegetables.
8. One-egg ranchero with corn tortilla.
9. Cooked rice with butter.

10. Steamed sweet potato with butter. Sweet potatoes are also good cold. They taste like candy.
11. One cup of popped corn.
12. My favorite quick breakfast is leftover rice heated with grated carrots, frozen peas, frozen lima beans, and butter.

Health-Promoting Eating Habits

Regardless of which Food Plan you're on, be sure to observe the following general health-promoting eating habits:

1. Chew each mouthful of food at least twenty times.
2. Do not wash foods down with liquids.
3. If you drink liquids during the meal, take small sips, and only when there is no food in your mouth.
4. Drink most of your liquids between meals.
5. Consume portion sizes you feel you can safely digest.
6. If you are emotionally upset or disturbed, eat smaller portions and chew more.
7. Do not overcook your food.
8. At each meal consume as much raw food as you do cooked.
9. Rather than eating large meals less often, consume smaller meals more often.
10. Examine each meal and snack from the viewpoint, "Does any part of this meal upset my body chemistry?"

These suggestions will lessen the body chemistry insult from your food habits and facilitate a more efficient digestion, assimilation, and utilization of nutrients. In addition, you will be supporting your body's ability to rebalance its chemistry after other lifestyle insults. Finally, your response to appropriate medical care will be enhanced.

Recipes

Appetizers

GARBANZO APPETIZER PATÉ

2 cups cooked garbanzo
  beans (chick peas),
  drained
3 tablespoons red wine
  vinegar
6 tablespoons olive oil
1/4 teaspoon cumin
Salt and pepper to taste
1/4 cup green pepper, minced
1/4 cup red pepper or
  pimiento, minced
2 tablespoons green onion,
  minced

In a food processor or
blender, combine garbanzo
beans, vinegar, oil, cumin,
and salt and pepper to taste.
Blend until well puréed.
Transfer to mixing bowl and
stir in green and red peppers
and green onion. Chill 4
hours. Serve with chilled raw
strips of peppers, carrots, jicama, celery, cucumbers,
and pita bread wedges, if desired. Makes about 2 cups.

SPLIT PEA-CURRY DIP

1/2 cup dried split peas
1 1/2 cups water
2 tablespoons butter
2 tablespoons onions,
  chopped
1/2 cup carrot, sliced
3/4 teaspoon curry powder

Cook peas until well done,
about 1 1/2 hours. If necessary, add more water to prevent burning. Allow excess
water to cook off. Cool. (Peas
should be the consistency of
applesauce.) Sauté onions
and carrots in butter over low
heat. Stir into split peas. Add
curry powder. Blend mixture
until carrots are well mashed.
Mixture will thicken as it
cools. Serve as a dip for raw
vegetables. Makes about 1
cup.

LUNCHEON SALAD with AVOCADO DRESSING

1 small sweet white onion,
  quartered and thinly
  sliced
1 green pepper, diced
1 small zucchini, diced
1 package (10 ounces) frozen
  cut corn, thawed and well

drained, or 2 ears fresh corn, kernels removed

1 cup cooked chick peas, drained

1 large tomato, chopped

1 small bunch coriander, chopped

Fresh ground pepper to taste

12 ounces assorted greens (any combination of lettuces, turnip greens, beet greens, dandelion greens, or spinach)

Avocado slices for garnish (optional)

AVOCADO DRESSING

1 ripe avocado, peeled and cut into chunks

2 tablespoons cider vinegar

Juice of one fresh lemon or lime

1 clove garlic, minced

$1/2$ teaspoon ground cumin

$1/2$ teaspoon chili powder

1 cup vegetable or tomato juice

Place avocado, vinegar, lime juice, garlic, cumin, and chili powder in a blender and process to purée. Add $3/4$ cup vegetable juice and blend until smooth.

In a large salad bowl, combine onion, green pepper, zucchini, corn, chick peas, tomato, and coriander. Sprinkle with ground pepper to taste. Add greens to salad bowl, add dressing, and toss well before serving. Makes 6 main-course servings.

ORIENTAL SALAD

1 tablespoon safflower oil

1 red pepper, sliced

1 green pepper, sliced

1 clove garlic, peeled

4 scallions, sliced

2 tablespoons soy sauce

$1/2$ cup (about 2 ounces) snow peas, washed, trimmed, and steamed

1 cup (about 3 ounces) sliced mushrooms

1 cup (about a handful) bean sprouts

1 soy bean curd, cubed

2 cups shredded lettuce or Chinese cabbage.

DRESSING

2 tablespoons water

2 tablespoons dry white wine

2 tablespoons soy sauce

$1/2$ teaspoon minced garlic

$1/2$ teaspoon minced ginger root or 1 teaspoon ground ginger

Heat oil in skillet or wok. Add peppers and garlic. Stir-fry 30 seconds. Add scallions and soy sauce. Stir and remove from heat. Cool. In a large bowl combine stir-fried ingredients, snow peas, mushrooms, sprouts, bean curd, and greens.

To make dressing, combine ingredients in a saucepan over medium heat. Stir. Bring to a boil and cook for 3 minutes. Cool. Pour over salad. Toss well. Serves 4.

MOLDED CHICKEN SALAD

3 cups cooked rice
2 cups cooked chicken, chopped
1 cup cooked green peas
1 cup celery, chopped
1/2 cup green onions (including tops), thinly sliced
1/4 cup pimientos, chopped
2 envelopes unflavored gelatin
1/2 cup double-strength chicken broth (cold)
2/3 cup mayonnaise
1 tablespoon lemon juice
2 teaspoons salt
1 teaspoon seasoned pepper

In a large mixing bowl combine rice, chicken, peas, celery, onions, and pimientos. Soften gelatin in broth; heat to dissolve; and combine with mayonnaise, lemon juice, salt, and pepper. Add to rice mixture and mix thoroughly.

Spoon into a 1 1/2-quart mold or individual molds. Chill until set. Unmold onto salad greens, if desired. Makes 6–8 servings.

DILL DRESSING

2 cups mayonnaise
4 teaspoons dill weed or 1/4 cup fresh dill, chopped
1/4 cup white vinegar
2 1/2 tablespoons prepared mustard

Place mayonnaise in a bowl and beat in dill, vinegar, and mustard, in that order. Beat with beater until fluffy. Let stand and chill. Serve at room temperature. Makes about 2 1/2 cups.

VEGETABLE SALAD with ARTICHOKE DRESSING

12 ounces cauliflower, cored and broken into very small flowerets

1 can (13 ¾ ounces)
    artichoke hearts, drained
    (reserve 5 hearts for
    dressing)

1 small red onion, thinly
    sliced

1 green pepper, thinly sliced

2 celery ribs, thinly sliced

1 can (3¼ ounces) pitted
    ripe olives, rinsed,
    drained, and sliced

12 ounces assorted greens
    (any combination of
    escarole, romaine, curly
    endive, dandelion greens,
    radicchio, or arugula) torn
    into pieces

1 can (6½ ounces) tuna in
    water, drained and flaked

8 ounces cherry tomatoes,
    halved

ARTICHOKE DRESSING

3 tablespoons (⅙ cup) olive
    oil

1 tablespoon balsamic or red
    wine vinegar

1 small clove garlic, minced

1 teaspoon dried oregano
    leaves

¼ teaspoon ground
    coriander

5 artichoke hearts, broken
    into pieces

½ cup dry white wine or
    lemon juice

Steam cauliflower until tender, but still crisp. Drain well. Place oil, vinegar, garlic, oregano, and coriander in blender with five artichoke hearts, broken into pieces, and the wine; process until smooth. Combine onion, green pepper, celery, olives, and remaining artichoke hearts, broken into pieces, in large salad bowl. Toss with greens, tuna, cauliflower, tomatoes, and ground pepper to taste. Spoon artichoke dressing over; toss well. Serves 6.

FRENCH VINAIGRETTE

½ cup safflower oil

2 tablespoons olive oil

3 tablespoons lemon juice

¾ teaspoon dry mustard

¼ teaspoon white pepper

¼ to ½ teaspoon dried
    tarragon, crushed

½ teaspoon coarse salt or ¼
    teaspoon regular salt

1 clove garlic, finely minced
    or pressed

Mix all ingredients in a blender. Serve cold over salad. Makes about 1 cup.

HERBED FRENCH DRESSING

1 tablespoon salt
1 teaspoon leaf oregano
1 teaspoon basil
1 teaspoon leaf tarragon
1 teaspoon onion powder
$1/2$ teaspoon garlic powder
$1/2$ teaspoon powdered
    mustard
$1/8$ teaspoon pepper
1 cup oil
$1/4$ cup cider vinegar
5 tablespoons lemon juice

Combine salt, oregano, basil, tarragon, onion powder, garlic powder, mustard, pepper, and oil. Let stand at least 1 hour. Add vinegar and lemon juice. Beat well with rotary beater. Makes about $1^1/3$ cups.

Soups

HOT CARROT SOUP

2 tablespoons butter
$3^1/2$ cups chicken broth
1 onion, minced
2 cloves garlic, chopped
$1/2$ teaspoon thyme

12 medium carrots, diced
2 medium potatoes, diced
2 stalks celery, diced
1 bay leaf
3 sprigs parsley
$1/4$ teaspoon pepper

Melt the butter in a medium-sized pot. Add the broth, onion, garlic, thyme, carrots, potatoes, celery, bay leaf, parsley, and pepper; simmer until vegetables are tender. Purée ingredients through a food mill or in a food processor. Serves 6.

TOMATO-VEGETABLE SOUP

6 cups tomato juice
4 tablespoons shredded
    carrot
4 tablespoons shredded
    celery
4 tablespoons shredded
    chives
1 large onion
1 small green pepper
$1/4$ teaspoon basil
$1/4$ teaspoon pepper

Bring ingrdients to boil in a pot. Reduce flame. Simmer 15 minutes till vegetables are tender. Serves 8.

ASPARAGUS SOUP

2 cups water
24 fresh asparagus spears
    (reserve tips), sliced
1 cup green onion, chopped
1 teaspoon fresh lemon juice
1/2 teaspoon garlic, finely
    chopped
White pepper, freshly
    ground
1 tablespoon whole wheat
    pastry flour or arrowroot
1 egg yolk
2 tablespoons fresh parsley,
    chopped
Herb or vegetable salt (to
    taste)

Heat water in a heavy 4-quart saucepan. Add asparagus (excluding tips), green onion, lemon juice, and garlic. Cover and cook until asparagus is tender-crisp, about 5–10 minutes. Season with pepper. Remove from heat and stir in flour or arrowroot. Place over low heat, stirring constantly. Reduce heat to very low and simmer 10 minutes. Transfer mixture to processor or blender in batches and puree (or press through fine strainer). Return puree to saucepan and set aside.

Steam asparagus tips until tender-crisp (about 5 minutes) and add them to the soup.

Remove approximately 1/2 cup of the soup broth to a small bowl. Add the egg yolk, mix, and return to pot. Stir in parsley and simmer (do not boil) over a low flame. Season with herb or vegetable salt. Serve hot or chilled. Serves 4.

Main Courses

POACHED FISH with ALMONDS

1/2 cup butter
1/2 cup lemon juice
2 tablespoons fresh or dried
    dill seed or fennel
1/4 teaspoon salt
1/4 teaspoon black pepper
1 pound fillet of sole,
    flounder, perch, or
    haddock
2/3 cup whole or slivered
    almonds

Heat wok or large skillet over a medium flame and melt

butter. Place lemon juice, dill, salt, and pepper in wok. Stir to blend. Place fish fillets in sauce. Spoon sauce over to cover fish. Reduce heat to low and poach, covered, 6 or 7 minutes or until fish flakes easily with fork. Remove fish to hot platter and spoon sauce over. Sprinkle almonds over top. Makes 4 to 6 servings.

MAIN COURSE SALAD

2 cups cooked cannellini, chick peas, or kidney beans (about 1 cup dry), drained, or 1 can (about 1 pound) cannellini, chick peas, or kidney beans, rinsed and drained
1 can (6 1/2 ounces) solid white tuna packed in spring water, drained and flaked
1/2 medium red pepper, halved lengthwise, seeded, then sliced crosswise into 1/4-inch strips (about 3/4 cup)
1/4 cup red onion, finely chopped
2 tablespoons fresh parsley, chopped
2 tablespoons fresh basil, chopped
Lettuce (optional)

DRESSING

3 tablespoons red-wine vinegar
1/4 teaspoon dry mustard
Freshly ground pepper
1/4 cup olive oil

Combine beans, tuna, pepper strips, onion, parsley, and basil in a medium-sized bowl. In a small bowl, stir together the vinegar, dry mustard, and pepper; next, add the olive oil in a slow stream, beating constantly. Pour dressing over bean mixture. Toss lightly to combine. Serve as is or on a bed of lettuce. Serves 2.

BAKED FISH SOUFFLÉ

2 pounds fresh or frozen fish fillets (if frozen, let thaw and drain)
1 1/4 teaspoons salt
1/4 teaspoon ground black pepper
3 egg whites
1/3 cup mayonnaise
1 tablespoon pickle relish

3 tablespoons scallions or
chives, chopped
1 tablespoon parsley,
chopped
2 drops Tabasco sauce

Preheat oven to 425° F. Place
fish fillets in lightly greased,
shallow, oven-to-table baking
pan. Sprinkle fish with 1 teaspoon salt and pepper. Place
in oven and bake 10 minutes.

Next, in a medium bowl,
beat the egg whites until stiff
peaks form. Blend in mayonnaise, relish, scallions and
parsley. Stir in the remaining
1/4 teaspoon salt and Tabasco
sauce.

Remove the fish from oven
and spread the egg white-
mayonnaise mixture on top,
covering completely. Return
to oven and continue baking
for 10 to 15 minutes until
topping is well puffed and
the fish flakes easily with a
fork. Makes 6 servings.

ONION-TOFU STIR-FRY

3 tablespoons oil
2 medium sweet red onions
(about 4 cups) sliced into
1/4-inch-thick rings
1 medium green pepper, cut
into strips

1 pound tofu, cut into cubes
1/2 cup water chestnuts,
sliced
2 tablespoons soy sauce
2 tablespoons sherry or
lemon juice
1 teaspoon cornstarch or
arrowroot
Salt and pepper (to taste)
Sesame seeds

Heat oil in a deep skillet or
wok. Add the onions and
green pepper and stir-fry
about 2 minutes. Carefully
stir in the tofu and water
chestnuts. Mix the soy sauce
with the sherry and corn-
starch and add to the skillet.
Cover and simmer 4–5 min-
utes or until heated through,
stirring occasionally. Season
to taste with salt and pepper.
Sprinkle with sesame seeds.
Serve with steamed rice.
Makes 3 to 4 servings.

SHRIMP and GREEN BEAN STIR-FRY

1 tablespoon oil
6–8 ounces raw shrimp,
peeled, de-veined, and cut
in half lengthwise
1 cup celery, diagonally
sliced
1/2 cup onion, sliced

1 cup green beans,
  diagonally sliced
1/2 cup chicken broth
1 teaspoon cornstarch
1/4 teaspoon salt
1 tablespoon soy sauce
2 cups hot cooked rice

In wok or skillet, heat the oil until very hot. Add shrimp and stir-fry 1 minute. Add the celery, onion, green beans, and 2 tablespoons of the broth. Cover and simmer 1 1/2 minutes. Remove cover and stir once. Blend the cornstarch, salt, and soy sauce with the remaining broth. Stir into the shrimp mixture. Cook and stir about 1 minute or until sauce is slightly thickened. Serve at once over rice. Serves 2.

POACHED SALMON with MUSHROOM SAUCE

1 cup fresh mushrooms
  (about 1/4 pound), sliced
1/2 cup onion, finely
  chopped
1 small clove garlic, minced
2 tablespoons softened
  butter
4 salmon steaks (about 1/2
  pound each)

1 can (10 3/4 ounces) chicken
  broth
1/2 cup Chablis or other dry
  white wine
1 large bay leaf
2 tablespoons cornstarch

In a skillet, sauté the mushrooms, onion, and garlic in butter until tender. Place the salmon steaks in the skillet. Add the broth (reserving 1/4 cup), wine, and bay leaf. Cover and bring to a boil. Reduce heat to low and simmer for 15 minutes. Discard the bay leaf and remove fish to heated platter.

Mix the cornstarch with the reserved broth and gradually blend into the mushroom mixture in the skillet. Cook, stirring until thickened. Spoon over fish. Serves 4.

Vegetables

VEGETABLE PLATTER with ANCHOVY-CAPER SAUCE

8 small red potatoes
12 ounces carrots, cut into
  1-inch pieces

4 large celery stalks, cut into
   3-inch-long pieces
1 medium-sized bunch
   broccoli, cut into flowerets
8 hard-boiled eggs, cut in
   half
2 medium-sized tomatoes,
   cut into wedges
1/4 cup walnuts, coarsely
   chopped
1 1/2-ounce can anchovy
   fillets (reserve 4 for sauce),
   chopped

ANCHOVY-CAPER SAUCE

4 anchovy fillets
1/3 cup safflower oil
1/4 cup cider vinegar
1 tablespoon capers,
   chopped

In a small bowl, mash 4 anchovies into a paste. Add oil, vinegar, and capers, and stir together until well blended.

Cut the potatoes in half, steam, and cool. Once cool, place potatoes in a large bowl, and pour two-thirds of the anchovy-caper sauce over. With a rubber spatula, stir gently to cover the potatoes with sauce. Cover and refrigerate. Cover the remaining anchovy-caper sauce

and refrigerate; it will be used later.

Lightly steam carrots, broccoli, and celery. Add to potato mixture, stir until well-coated, and refrigerate one hour to blend flavors.

Arrange marinated vegetable mixture, egg halves, and tomato wedges on a large platter. Pour remaining anchovy-caper sauce over eggs and tomatoes. Sprinkle chopped anchovies and walnuts over vegetable platter. Serves 8.

LOTSA VEGETABLES

1 1/2 cups water
1 chicken bouillon cube
3/4 cup onion, chopped
3/4 cup celery, chopped
1/4 cup soy sauce
1 teaspoon garlic salt
4 mushrooms, sliced
2 small zucchini, thinly
   sliced
2 cups broccoli, chopped
1 cup bean sprouts
1 cup water chestnuts, sliced

In a skillet or large pan, bring the water and bouillon cube to boil. Add the onion, celery, soy sauce, and garlic salt. Cover and continue boiling 5 minutes. Next, add the mushrooms, zucchini, broccoli, bean sprouts, and water chestnuts. Stir until the mixture comes to a full boil, then reduce the flame to low and simmer gently, uncovered. Stir frequently, for about 15 minutes or until the vegetables are tender-crisp and the liquid is reduced. Serves 4.

VEGETABLE CURRY

1/4 cup apricot kernel or
  sesame oil
1 large onion, minced
3 tablespoons coconut,
  grated
2 cloves garlic, minced
1 1/2 tablespoons curry
  powder
1 teaspoon vegetable-mineral
  salt
2 pounds assorted raw
  vegetables, cut or diced
  into bite-sized pieces (any
  combination of broccoli,
  zucchini, kohlrabi,
  turnips, potatoes, celery,
  carrots, or cabbage will
  do)
3 tomatoes, peeled and diced
1 1/2 cups water or meat
  broth

Heat the oil in a large, heavy skillet. Add the onion, coconut, and garlic, and sauté until the onion is soft. Blend in the curry powder and vegetable-mineral salt, and stir over a low flame for about a minute. Add the vegetables, tomatoes, and water, and bring to a boil. Reduce the heat and simmer, stirring occasionally, until the vegetables are tender. Serves 4–6.

AVOCADO HALVES with CURRIED VEGETABLE FILLING and CREAM SAUCE

4 medium-sized avocados,
  halved
1 1/2 cups pecans

CURRIED VEGETABLE FILLING

3 tablespoons butter, melted
2 cups small mushrooms,
  de-stemmed (reserve
  stems) and halved
1 onion, chopped
1 clove garlic, minced
1–3 teaspoons curry powder
  (to taste)
1 cup broccoli, finely
  chopped

1 cup cauliflower, finely
chopped
1 cup eggplant, cut into
$1/2$-inch cubes
$1/4$ cup vegetable stock
1 cup shelled peas

CREAM SAUCE

3 tablespoons butter
3 tablespoons flour, brown
rice flour, or arrowroot
$1^1/_2$ cups coconut milk

Melt butter in a frying pan
and sauté mushroom stems,
onion, garlic, and curry.
When onion is transparent,
add broccoli, cauliflower,
eggplant, mushrooms, and
vegetable stock. Cover and
simmer over low heat until
vegetables are tender. During
the last 5 minutes of cooking,
add the peas.

For cream sauce, melt the
butter in a pan, add flour,
and cook over low heat for 2
minutes, stirring constantly.
Very slowly, add the coconut
milk, whisking or stirring
constantly. Simmer gently,
frequently stirring, for 10
minutes.

Place the warm, cooked
vegetables in prepared avocado halves. Cover lightly
with cream sauce and sprinkle with pecans. Bake 15
minutes at 350° F. Serve im-
mediately. Fills 8 medium-
sized avocado halves.

Glossary

adrenal glands: two glands in the upper back part of the abdomen that produce and secrete vital hormones

adrenalin (epinephrine): one of the hormones secreted by the adrenal glands

antacid: a substance that relieves excess acidity, such as stomach acidity

anorexia: lack of desire for food

antibody: a substance produced in the blood of an individual that is capable of producing a specific immunity to a specific foreign body such as a virus, bacteria, or allergen

artery: a vessel carrying blood from the heart

basal metabolism: the lowest level of metabolism

biochemistry: the chemistry of live tissue

body chemistry: the functioning of the body systems that depends upon the body's chemical balance, which depends in turn upon balanced mineral relationships

bone reabsorption: the breakdown and dissolving of bone in the process of remodeling

bone remodeling: the process of bone breakdown and formation that is responsible for growth, maintenance, and repair of bone tissue

buffer systems: those systems in our body that preserve the balance of acidity and alkalinity of a solution

cataract: a cloudiness in the lens of the eye

chelator: an agent used to remove a substance

corticosteroids: drugs sometimes used in the treatment of arthritis or asthma; they resemble adrenal hormones

cortical bone: the hard, dense bone that forms the outer shell of all bones

covalent bond: a chemical bond formed by the sharing of electron pairs

debility: weakness

degenerative disease: a deterioration of tissue with loss of function and eventual destruction of the particular tissue cells

dowager's hump: outward curvature of the upper spine caused by collapsing of the vertebrae, found primarily in older women

emulsifying agent: an agent used in food to solidify parts of the substance

endocrine glands: glands, such as pituitary, thyroid, and adrenal, that secrete their hormones into the bloodstream

enzyme: a protein that accelerates specific chemical reactions, but does not itself undergo any change during the reaction; a biochemical catalyst; digestive enzymes are produced by glands and organs to break down complex carbohydrates into simple sugars, fats or lipids into fatty acids, and glycerol, glycerides, and protein into amino acids

estrogen: the hormone responsible for the development and maintenance of female sexual characteristics and reproductive functions in women; the ovaries produce estrogen in women and the testes produce small amounts of estrogen in men

extracellular: outside the cell

gonad: a sex gland; the ovary or testicle

homeostasis (homeostatic mechanism): stability of all body functions at normal levels; a mechanism used by the body to maintain a stable chemical internal environment, despite external changes; this is accomplished in large part by the hormones

hormone: a chemical produced by a gland, secreted into the bloodstream, and affecting the function of distant cells and organs

hyperglycemia: excessive sugar in the blood

hypoglycemia: too little sugar in the blood

hypothalamus: a specialized portion of the brain, the coordinating center of the endocrine system; it receives and integrates messages from the central nervous system

immune complexes: antibodies are formed in our body as a protective mechanism; when these substances combine with a foreign invader such as a bacteria, virus, or food allergen, these complexes can cause problems in our body

immune system: the body's system that defends us against disease, composed primarily of white blood cells

insulin: a hormone produced in the cells of the pancreas; when secreted into the bloodstream, it permits the metabolism and utilization of sugar; an insufficient secretion of insulin causes hyperglycemia; too much insulin secretion causes hypoglycemia

intracellular: inside the cell

ionically bonded: bonded together by an electrical charge

lactation: the secretion of milk from the mother's breast

malaise: the feeling of being sick

membrane: a thin layer of tissue

metabolism: the process by which foods are transformed into basic elements that can be utilized by the body for energy or growth

multiple sclerosis: deposits of abnormal connective tissue in the central nervous system

osteoarthritis: a form of arthritis associated with bone and cartilage degeneration

osteomalacia: softening of the bone

osteopenia: a reduction in overall bone mass to a level below normal, but still above that associated with fracturing

osteoporosis: loss of bone or skeletal tissue, producing brittleness or softness of bone

pancreas: a large gland, six to eight inches long, lying crosswise in the upper posterior portion of the abdomen; it secretes enzymes into the intestines to digest food, and it manufactures insulin that is secreted into the bloodstream

parathormone: the hormone secreted by the parathyroid glands

parathyroid glands: four small endocrine glands located in the neck behind the thyroid gland; they secrete the hormone that controls calcium and phosphorus secretion

periodontal disease: disease of the tissues, including the gums that surround the teeth

peptic ulcer: an ulcer of the stomach, duodenum, or lower end of the esophagus

pH: a symbol denoting acidity or alkalinity; a solution of pH 7 is neutral, below 7 is acidic, above 7 is alkaline

pituitary gland: an important endocrine gland located at the base of the brain; its hormones regulate growth and seem to control the secretions of other endocrine glands

post-menopausal: after menstruation has stopped

pseudofracture: a condition in which new bone is formed at the site of an old injury to a bone

psoriasis: a non-contagious, chronic skin disease with reddish silvery patches located on the chest, knees, and elbows; it may come and go throughout the patient's entire life

rickets: a disease occurring chiefly in children, caused by lack of vitamin D; it is evidenced in marked cases by bone deformities such as bowlegs and funnel chest

systemic: referring to a condition or disease involving the entire body, as opposed to a localized condition

thyroid gland: the endocrine gland, located in the front of the neck, which regulates body metabolism; it secretes a hormone known as thyroxin

thrombosis: formation of a blood clot

thyroxin: the hormone manufactured by the thyroid gland containing large quantities of iodine

trabecular bone: the porous, spongy bone that lines the bone marrow cavity and is surrounded by cortical bone

vein: a blood vessel that transports blood from the tissues back to the heart

venous thrombosis: blood clotting in the veins

vertebra: one of the bones forming the spinal column

Bibliography

Chapter 1. Holey Bones
Appleton, Nancy. *Lick the Sugar Habit*. Garden City Park, New York: Avery Publishing Group Inc., 1988.

Fromer, Margot Joan. *Osteoporosis*. New York: Pocket Books, 1986.

Hausman, Patricia. *The Calcium Bible*. New York: Warner Books, 1985.

Kamen, Betty, and Kamen, Si. *Osteoporosis: What It Is, How to Prevent It, How to Stop It*. New York: Pinnacle Books Inc., 1984.

Mayes, Kathleen. *Osteoporosis: Brittle Bones and the Calcium Crisis*. Santa Barbara, California: Pennant Books, 1986.

Notelovitz, Morris, and Ware, Marsha. *Stand Tall.* New York: Bantam Books, 1985.

Chapter 2. Your Body Chemistry

THE ENDOCRINE SYSTEM

Blomberg, B. M., et al. "Urinary Estrogens and Neutral Oxosteroids in the South African Bantu with and without Hepatic Disease." *Journal of Endocrinology* 17 (1958): 182.

Ettinger, B. "Thyroid Supplements: Effect on Bone Mass." *Western Journal of Medicine* 136 (1984): 473.

Kamen, Betty, and Kamen, Si. *Osteoporosis: What It Is, How to Prevent It, How to Stop It.* New York: Pinnacle Books Inc., 1984.

Mayes, Katherine. *Osteoporosis: Brittle Bones and the Calcium Crisis.* Santa Barbara, California: Pennant Books, 1986.

Notelovitz, Morris, and Ware, Marsha. *Stand Tall.* New York: Bantam Books, 1985.

MINERAL RELATIONSHIPS

Appleton, Nancy. *Lick the Sugar Habit.* Garden City Park, New York: Avery Publishing Group Inc., 1988.

Page, Melvin E., and Abrams, H. Leon, Jr. *Your Body Is Your Best Doctor.* New Canaan, Connecticut: Keats Publishing, 1972.

ACID-ALKALINE BALANCE

Brazel, Uriel S. "Osteoporosis in Young Men." *Archives of Internal Medicine* 142 (November 1982): 2079-2080.

Dawson-Hughes, Bess, Seligson, Frances H., and Hughes, Virginia A. "Effects of Calcium Carbonate and Hydroxyapatite on Zinc and Iron Retention in Postmenopausal Women." *American Journal of Clinical Nutrition* 44 (1986): 83–88.

Lemann, Jacob, Jr., et al. "Studies of the Mechanism by which Chronic Metabolic Acidosis Augments Urinary Calcium Excretion in Man." *Journal of Clinical Investigation* 4, 1318 (1967).

Morter, M. T., Jr. *Correlative Urinalysis: The Body Knows Best.* Rogers, Arkansas: B.E.S.T. Research Inc., 1987.

Wackman, A., and Bernstein, D. D. "Diet and Osteoporosis." *Lancet* (May 4, 1968): 958–959.

OTHER DISEASES

McCain, Toni, and Haussler, Mark R. "Experimental Diabetes Reduces Circulating 1, 25-Dihydroxyvitamin D in the Rat." *Science* 196 (June 1977): 1452–1454.

Chapter 3. What's Eating You?

MENTAL AND PHYSICAL DISTRESS

Allen, Pat. *Conversational Rape.* Newport Beach, California: Pat Allen Programs, 1987.

Foundation of Inner Peace. *The Course in Miracles.* Farmingdale, New York: 1980.

Kübler-Ross, Elizabeth. *On Death and Dying.* New York: Macmillan Publishing Company, 1969.

Rosenberg, J. L., Rand, M. L., and Asay, Diane. *Body, Self & Soul.* Atlanta, Georgia: Humanistics Limited, Humanics New Age, 1985.

SUGAR

Holl, Marita G., and Allen, Lindsay H. "Sucrose Ingestion Insulin Response and Mineral Metabolism in Humans." *Journal of Nutrition* 117 (1987): 1229–1233.

Lemann, J. "Evidence that Glucose Ingestion Inhibits Net Renal Tubular Reabsorption of Calcium and Magnesium in Man." *Journal of Laboratory and Clinical Medicine* 70 (1967): 236–245.

Orr, J. B. "The Importance of the Mineral Elements in the Maintenance of Health." *British Medical Journal* 504, Vol. II (Sept. 20, 1924): 504–508.

Page, Melvin E., and Abrams, H. Leon, Jr. *Your Body Is Your Best Doctor*. New Canaan, Connecticut: Keats Publishing, 1972.

Schneider, Joseph Z. "The Calcium to Phosphorus Ratio as Related to Mineral Metabolism." *International Journal of Orthodontists* 16:3 (March 1930) 277–285.

DAIRY PRODUCTS
Abrahams, Guy E. "The Calcium Controversy." *Journal of Applied Nutrition* 34, no. 2 (1982): 69–73.

SALT
Shealey, Tom. "It's Time to Bone Up on Calcium." *Prevention* (Oct. 1985): 109–120.

Whittlesey, Marietta. *Killer Salt*. New York: Avon Books, 1978.

CAFFEINE
Heaney, Robert P., and Recker, Robert R. "Effects of Nitrogen, Phosphorus and Caffeine on Calcium Balance in Women." *Journal of Laboratory Clinical Medicine* 99 (1982): 46–55.

Hollingberg, P., and Massey, L. "Effect of Dietary Caffeine and Sucrose on Urinary Calcium Excretion in Adolescents." *Federal Protocol* 45 (1968): 375.

Massey, Linda K., and Wise, Kevin J. "The Effect of Dietary Caffeine on Urinary Secretion of Calcium, Magnesium, Sodium, and Potassium in Healthy Young Females." *Nutrition Research* 4 (1984): 43–50.

Yeh, James K., Aloia, John F., Semla, Halena M., and Chen, Shang Y. "Influence of Injected Caffeine on the Metabolism of Calcium and the Retention and Excretion of Sodium, Potassium, Phosphorus, Magnesium, Zinc, and Copper in Rats." *Journal of Nutrition* 116, no. 2 (Feb. 1986): 273–280.

TOBACCO

Bailey, Alan, Robinson, David, and Vessey, Martin. "Smoking and Age on Natural Menopause." *Lancet* (Oct. 1, 1977): 722.

Bhattacharyya, M. H., Whelton, B. D., Stern, P. H., and Peterson, D. P. "Cadmium Accelerates Bone Loss in Ovariectomized Mice and Fetal Rat Limb Bones in Culture." *Proceedings of the National Academy of Sciences* 85 (Nov. 1988): 8761–8765.

Daniell, Harry W., M. D. "Osteoporosis of the Slender Smoker." *Archives of Internal Medicine* 136 (March 1976): 298–304.

Harstad, Grace J. "Osteoporosis, You Can Prevent Brittle Bones If You Start Now." *Bestways* (March 1984): 48.

International Clinical Nutrition Review 7, no. 4 (Oct. 1987): 17.

Michnovicz, J. J., Hershcopf, R. J., Naganuna, H., et al. "Increased 2-Hydroxylation of Oestradoil as a Possible Mechanism for the Anti-Oestrogenic Effect of Cigarette

Smoking." *New England Journal of Medicine* 35 (1986): 1305–1309.

ALCOHOL

Dalen, N., and Lamke, B. "Bone Mineral Losses in Alcoholics." *Acta Ortho Scandinavia* 47 (1976): 469–471.

"It's Time to Bone Up on Calcium." *Prevention* (Oct. 1985): 109–120.

McDonald, Janet T., and Margeh, Sheldon. "Wine versus Ethanol in Human Nutrition, Calcium, Phosphorus, and Magnesium Balance." *American Journal of Clinical Nutrition* 32 (April 1979): 823–833.

Saville, D. D. "Changes in Bone Mass with Age and Alcoholism." *Journal of Bone Joint Surgery* 47A (1965): 492.

OVERCOOKED FOOD

Pottenger, Francis M., Jr. *Pottenger's Cats*. LaMesa, California: Price Pottenger Nutritional Foundation, 1983.

Steggerda, F. R., and Mitchell, H. H. "Variability in the Calcium Metabolism and Calcium Requirements of Adult Human Subjects." Department of Zoology and Physiology and Division of Animal Nutrition, University of Illinois, Urbana, Nov. 1945.

PROTEIN

Allen, L. H., Bartlett, R. S., and Block, G. P. "Reduction of Renal Calcium Absorption in Man by Consumption of Dietary Protein." *Journal of Nutrition* 109 (1979): 1345–1350.

Allen, L. H., Block, G. D., Wood, R. N., and Bryce, G. F. "The Role of Insulin and Parathyroid Hormone in the Protein-Induced Calciuria of Man." *Nutrition Research* 1 (1981): 11.

Allen, L. H., Oddoye, E. A., and Margen, S. "Protein Induced Hypercalciuria: A Long-Term Study." *American Journal of Clinical Nutrition* 32 (1979): 711–749.

Harstad, Grace J. "Osteoporosis: You Can Prevent Brittle Bones if You Get Started Now." *Bestways* (March 1984): 48.

Margen, S., et al. "Studies in Calcium Metabolism. The Calciuretic Effect of Dietary Protein." *American Journal of Clinical Nutrition* 27 (1974): 584–589.

Mazess, R. B., and Mather, W. "Bone Mineral Content of North Alaskan Eskimos." *American Journal of Clinical Nutrition* 27 (1984): 916–925.

Robbins, John. *Diet for a New America*. Walpole, New Hampshire: Stillpoint Publishing, 1987.

PHOSPHORUS
Bell, R. R., Draper, H. H., Lzend, D. Y. M., et al. "Physiological Responses of Human Adults to Foods Containing Phosphate Additives." *Journal of Nutrition* 104 (1977): 42.

Draper, Harold H., and Bell, R. Raines. "Nutrition and Osteoporosis." *Advances in Nutritional Research*. New York: Plenum Press, 1979.

Ellinger, R. H. "Phosphates in Food Processing." *Handbook of Food Additives*. Cleveland, Ohio: CRC Press (1972): 617–780.

Lotz, M. E., Tisman, Elias, and Baxter, Frederic, C. "Evidence for a Phosphorus Depletion Syndrome in Man." *New England Journal of Medicine* 278 (1968): 409–415.

CALCIUM SUPPLEMENTS
Abraham, Guy E. "The Calcium Controversy." *Journal of Applied Nutrition* 34, no. 2 (1982): 69–73.

Allen, L. H. "Calcium Bioavailability and Absorption: A Review." *American Journal of Clinical Nutrition* 35 (April 1982): 186–187.

Bailey, D. A., Martin, A. D., Houstin, C. S., and Howie, J. L. "Physical Activity, Nutrition, Bone Loss, and Osteoporosis." *Australian Journal of Science Medicine in Sports* 18, no. 3 (Sept. 1986): 3–8.

Nelas, L., Christiansen, C., and Rodbro, P. "Calcium Supplementation and Postmenopausal Bone Loss." *British Journal of Medicine* 289 (Oct. 27, 1984): 1103–1105.

Riis, Bente, Thompson, Karsten, and Christiansen, Claus. "Does Calcium Supplementation Prevent Postmenopausal Bone Loss?" *New England Journal of Medicine* 316, no. 4 (Jan. 27, 1987): 173–177.

Snedeker, Suzanne M., Smith, Sylvia A., and Greger, J. L. "Effect of Dietary Calcium and Phosphorus Levels on the Utilization of Iron, Copper, and Zinc by Adult Males." *Journal of Nutrition* 112 (1982): 136–143.

University of California at Berkeley, *Wellness Letter* 3, no. 12 (Sept. 1987): 1.

OVER-THE-COUNTER AND PRESCRIPTION DRUGS

Adinoff, Allen P., and Hollister, J. Roger. "Steroid-Induced Fractures and Bone Loss in Patients with Asthma." *New England Journal of Medicine* 309 (August 4, 1983): 265–268.

Allen, L. H. "Calcium Absorption and Bioavailability: A Review." *American Journal of Clinical Nutrition* 35 (1982): 783–808.

Gilman, Alfred Goodman, Goodman, L. S., Rall, Theodore W., and Murad, F. *The Pharmacological Basis of Therapeu-*

tics 7th Ed. New York: Macmillan Publishing Company, 1985: 1188.

Smith, Dorothy L. "Taking Medicines: Update on Aspirin." *Medical Update* x, no. 5 (Nov. 1986): 2.

Spencer, H., et al. "Effects of Small Doses of Aluminum-Containing Antacids on Calcium and Phosphorus Metabolism." *American Journal of Clinical Nutrition* 36 (1982): 32–40.

Spencer, Keith, and Kramer, Lois. "Antacid-Induced Calcium Loss." *Archives of Internal Medicine* 143, no. 4 (April 1983): 657–659.

Watts, Nelson B., and others. "Intermittant Cyclical Etidronate Treatment of Postmenopausal Osteoporosis." *New England Journal of Medicine* 323, no. 2 (July 12, 1990): 73–79.

FLUORIDATION
Draper, Harold, ed. *Advances in Nutritional Research*. New York: Plenum Press, 1979.

"Fluoridation—Good or Bad?" *Health Freedom News* (Jan. 1987): 35, 42, 44.

INTRAVENOUS FEEDING
Klein, G. L., et al. "Bone Disease Associated with Total Parenteral Nutrition." *Lancet* 15 (Nov. 15, 1980): 1041.

Wood, Richard J., Setrin, Michael D., and Rosenberg, Irwin H., M. D. "Calcium in Total Parenteral Nutrition: Effects of Amino Acids and Glucose in Rats." *American Journal of Clinical Nutrition* 40 (1984): 101–106.

HEAVY METALS
Brekhman I. I. *Man and Biologically Active Substances—The Effect of Drugs, Diet and Pollution on Health*. New York: Pergamon Press, 1980.

Mayo, G. H., Keiser, J. A., and Pao, K. K. "Aluminum Absorption and Distribution: Effects on the Parathyroid Hormone." *Science* 197 (1977): 1187–1189.

Silbergeld, E. K. "Experimental Studies of Lead Neurotoxicity at Low Dose." International Symposium organized by the *Clear* Charitable Trust and sponsored by Pura Foods, Ltd., May 10-12, 1982. United Kingdom.

Chapter 4. Balancing Act

EXERCISE

Ayalon, J., Simkin, A., Leichter, I., and Raefmann, S. "Dynamic Bone Loading Exercises of Post Menopausal Women." *Archives of Physical Medical Rehabilitation* 68, no. 5 (May 1987): 280–283.

Bailey, D. A., Martin, A. D., Houstin, C. S., and Howie, J. L. "Physical Activity, Nutrition, Bone Density, and Osteoporosis." *Australian Journal of Science Medicine in Sports* (Sept. 3–7, 1986).

Lane, N. E., Block, D. A., Jones, H. H., et al. "Long Distance Running, Bone Density and Osteoarthritis." *Journal of American Medical Association* 255, no. 9 (1986): 1147–1151.

Lawton, Grant. "Exercise, Energy and Body Integrity." *Complimentary Medicine* (Fall 1987).

Panusk, R. S., Schmidt, C., Caldwell, J. R., et al. "Is Running Associated with Degenerating Joint Disease?" *Journal of American Medical Association* 255, no. 9 (1986): 1152–1154.

Sinaki, Mehrsheed, McPhee, Malcolm C., Hodgson, Stephen F., et al. "Relationship Between Bone Mineral Density of Spine and Strength of Back Extensors in Healthy Post

Menopausal Women." *Mayo Clinic Proceedings* 61 (1986): 116.

Smith, D. M., Khairi, M.R.A., Norton, J., and Johnston, C. C., Jr. "Age and Activity Effects on Rate of Bone Mineral Loss." *Journal of Clinical Investigation* 58: 716.

Index

AUDIO CASSETTES

An extensive look at each of these subjects is available on tape cassettes.

LICK THE SUGAR HABIT—This tape is an introduction to the book. It explains, in detail, the body chemistry principle, mineral relationships, the endocrine system, enzymes, and what promotes infectious and degenerative diseases. (1 hour)

ALLERGIES—The subjects of this tape are allergies, what causes them, and how to eliminate them. Learn how foods to which you react can be reintroduced back into your diet. The subject of inhalant allergies is also explored. (1 hour)

OSTEOPOROSIS—You may be getting a reasonable amount of calcium in your diet, but, if you are eating abusive foods or upsetting your lifestyle in other ways, the calcium will not absorb as well. What you do not eat is more important than what you do eat. This tape tells how to look for symptoms and how to test for susceptibility to osteoporosis. (1 hour)

OBESITY—The newest research on what works and what doesn't is discussed. You will understand the relationship of allergies, addictions, and cravings to obesity. (1/2 hour) WOMEN/opposite side.

WOMEN—Premenstrual syndrome (P.M.S.), candida albicans (yeast infections), menses, menopause, and post menopausal problems are discussed on this tape. (1/2 hour) OBESITY/opposite side.

CHILDREN—The first subject on this tape is nutrition during pregnancy. Infants' and children's eating problems are then discussed, as well as children's allergies. Ideas to help teenagers eat nutritious foods end the tape. (1 hour)

ORDER FORM
BODY CHEMISTRY TEST KIT

This kit is used to determine if your minerals are in the correct relationship to each other and if your body chemistry is in balance. The kit includes solution to use for 250 tests, two test tubes, an eye dropper, a brush for cleaning test tubes, and the instruction book, *Monitoring Your Basic Health*. The book contains a section on what upsets body chemistry, suggestions on how to balance body chemistry, food plans, and a section on how to test for food allergies. pH paper to test for acid-alkalinity of the saliva is also included.

NAME: _____

ADDRESS: _____ APT: _____

CITY: _____

STATE: _____ ZIP: _____

1 kit	$20.00
Shipping	$ 1.50
Sales tax (California residents only)	$ 1.65

Make check payable to:

Nancy Appleton, Ph.D.
P.O. Box 3083
Santa Monica, CA 90403-3083

FOOD PREPARATION—Where and how to buy food, insecticides, fungicides, food irradiation, additives, vitamins, minerals, and how to prepare food so that it will not upset the body chemistry are discussed. (1 hour)

URINE AND PH TESTING—Information is given as to how to test for homeostasis of urine and saliva. Suggestions are given as to what causes upset body chemistry and how to help balance it. (1 hour)

NEW INFORMATION—Information from medical journals linking health, the medical field, and nutrition. (1 hour)

	One*	Two*	Three*	Four*
Price of tape	$ 6.00	$12.00	$15.00	$20.00
Sales Tax (Calif. only)	$ .50	$ .99	$ 1.24	$ 1.65
Shipping	$ 1.00	$ 1.25	$ 1.50	$ 1.75

	Five*	Six*	Seven*	Eight*
Price of tape	$25.00	$30.00	$35.00	$40.00
Sales Tax (Calif. only)	$ 2.06	$ 2.48	$ 2.89	$ 2.99
Shipping	$ 2.00	$ 2.00	$ 2.00	$ 2.00

*Specify which tape(s) you want. Make check payable to:

Nancy Appleton, Ph.D.
P.O. Box 3083
Santa Monica, CA 90403